Saving Very Premature Babies
Key Ethical Issues

To all the children with profound and multiple learning disabilities, their families, and those who educate and care for them daily.

For Books for Midwives:

Commissioning Editor: Mary Seager
Development Editor: Catherine Steers
Project Management: Ailsa Laing / Temple DPS
Design: George Ajayi

Angela Smith

Saving Very Premature Babies

Key Ethical Issues

Pauline Challinor Mifflin MA (Medical Ethics) Cert Ed
Freelance writer who worked in midwifery, social services and teaching. Head of Department in a school for children with severe learning disabilities.

BfM Books *for* Midwives

An Imprint of Elsevier Science

EDINBURGH LONDON NEW YORK OXFORD PHILADELPHIA ST LOUIS SYDNEY TORONTO 2003

ISBN 0 7506 5412 0

British Library Cataloguing in Publication Data
A catalogue record for this book is available from the British Library

Library of Congress Cataloging in Publication Data
A catalog record for this book is available from the Library of Congress

Notice
Medical knowledge is constantly changing. Standard safety precautions must be followed, but as new research and clinical experience broaden our knowledge, changes in treatment and drug therapy may become neccessary or appropriate. Readers are advised to check the most current product information provided by the manufacturer of each drug to be administered to verify the recommended dose, the method and duration of administration, and contraindications. It is the responsibility of the practitioner, relying on experience and knowledge of the patient, to determine dosages and the best treatment for each individual patient. Neither the Publisher nor the author assumes any liability for any injury and/or damage to persons or property arising from this publication.

The Publisher

The publisher's policy is to use **paper manufactured from sustainable forests**

Printed in China

Contents

Acknowledgements

Firstly, I would like to thank all the parents, teachers, medical staff and care workers for their help and comments; secondly, I would like to acknowledge the many children with profound and multiple learning disabilities whom I taught, because their daily struggles inspired me to write this book. Lastly, I thank my husband Brian, who was always ready to put another viewpoint, but was also a great source of positive encouragement when I needed a push!

1

Introduction

The rapid advance in neonatal technology now enables doctors to save many more premature babies than ever before. It is now possible to save babies born as early as 21 or 22 weeks' gestation, just over halfway through a normal pregnancy. This gives hope to many parents whose babies would have died a few years ago.

Julia Sommerfield (2001) describes one such baby, Justin Washington, who was born four months early. His mother had spent one month in the antenatal unit at an American hospital, in an effort to prevent his premature birth. He came into the world weighing 680 grams (1½ pounds), and spent the next four months in the intensive care unit on ventilation. During that time he developed a liver malfunction, an intestinal hernia and eye problems, all of which needed surgery. Six years later, Justin is a healthy, active child with no sign of his traumatic start to life. Thanks to the skill and dedication of medical staff, and the life-saving techniques now available, not only was his life saved, but he is able to live it to the full within a loving family environment. Naturally when this outcome is achieved, everyone rejoices with the parents, while doctors and nurses feel a deep sense of satisfaction in the part they were able to play.

Unfortunately, however, not all infants born very prematurely are so fortunate. Ironically, many of those who survive being born at such an early stage are left with severe mental and physical disabilities as a result of the very treatment that initially saved their lives. When this happens, it is natural that the medical teams who work so hard to save lives begin to question the wisdom of using such methods on such fragile infants. Parents, too, may sometimes feel that the price their child has to pay for merely living is far too high.

I was motivated to write this book because, as a teacher of children with special educational needs, my main area of work has been with pupils with profound and multiple learning disabilities. During the last decade or so, my colleagues and I have been struck by the increased intake into the school of these very severely mentally and physically impaired children, whose disabilities may include some or all of the following: blindness, deafness, gross and fine motor problems, hydrocephalus, speech disorders, chest and intestinal conditions, along with severe mental retardation. Many spend their entire lives confined to wheelchairs, unable to sit or stand unaided, and are completely dependent on others for all their everyday needs. Often they have little awareness of self or others.

Alongside this, but in direct contrast, the intake of pupils with conditions such as Down's Syndrome and spina bifida, which carry with them a far wider range of mental and physical abilities, has declined; and as we all know, many people suffering from such disabilities are capable of living fairly independent, happy and fulfilling lives. Allowing for the fact that a few of the children born with these conditions are now being integrated into mainstream schools, the main reason for this anomaly seems to be that these and other abnormalities are now detected by antenatal screening, and women are given the option of terminating their pregnancy. Approximately 92% of all cases of foetal abnormality diagnosed by amniocentesis in pregnancy now end in abortion, with the result that the number of these children in schools has decreased considerably over the past twenty years.

One of the things that intrigued me was that many of the children with the profound disabilities that I have described were born very prematurely, sometimes as early as twenty-two or twenty-three weeks of gestation, with extremely low birth weights. Following intensive and sometimes aggressive medical interventions to save or prolong their lives, they survive with extensive neurological damage and grow up with crippling mental and physical disabilities.

Do these rapid advances in both antenatal and neonatal technology mean that we have the means to phase out one set of abnormalities, only to be faced with another, potentially more serious set? What, if any, are the long-term implications of these breakthroughs for the child, the family and society in general?

My experience has shown me that while the families who care for them are, in the main, fiercely protective of these children, loving them just as much and sometimes even more than their more able siblings, the burden can become intolerable at times. Even when family members are loving and supportive of each other, their whole lives inevitably revolve around the needs of the multiply disabled child. Their problems will never diminish; they will probably increase as time goes by.

The education of these children poses many problems, but in many ways it is a learning experience for teachers and helpers too. I very quickly discovered that although all the children I worked with were profoundly mentally impaired, with few or no communication skills at all, some barely appearing to recognise even their parents, each child is distinctly individual. They have their own unique behaviours and needs, their own likes and dislikes. They have distinctive ways of making their feelings and needs known, and they act and react in many different ways.

Alongside the considerations about how crippling disabilities affect the lives of the children and their immediate families, issues can also be raised about how the lives of these children impinge on the lives of others in the wider community.

Some would question whether it is ethically justifiable, in the light of limited NHS resources, to use expensive technology for relatively few, high-risk cases; by diverting funds, more babies with less risk of severe impairment could be saved. Some would also question whether it is possible morally to justify saving these babies, only to send them home to families who then have to spend the rest of their lives struggling daily to live as normally as possible within a climate of dwindling health care resources and social services.

These questions bring into focus huge philosophical issues concerning the sanctity of life, the value and quality of life; whether every human being is a 'real person' and whether every individual has an intrinsic right to life, however badly disabled they may be.

Whatever their ethical stance on matters relating to the treatment of very premature babies, doctors and parents have certain legal obligations laid upon them which limit their actions and choices in relation to the care of the child. However, with rapid progress being made in medical science, advances in research and technology are presenting new problems for both the medical profession and the moral philosophers. This in turn highlights inadequacies in the legal framework when it is applied to such complex issues, prompting the current debate about whether or not the law needs to be reviewed.

Margaret Brazier (1992) considers two crucial areas of public concern: The growth in medical technology, which has given doctors greater power over life and death, and the fact that there is no longer a general consensus about the sanctity of life: when it begins, when it ends and whether every life is equally valuable.

According to David Woodrum (1998), a person in favour of the advances in neonatal care might argue:

> Neonatal intensive care is responsible for the survival of a significant number of infants who formerly would not have survived. This increased survival has been accomplished with an acceptable burden and without substantially increasing the population of handicapped children.

An opponent of the technology now available might consider that:

> Neonatal intensive care is a good example of medicine out of control. There is inappropriate use of technology by health care professional who are out of touch with patients and their families. The benefits of increased survival of high risk infants are outweighed by the associated burdens.

My intentions in writing this book were twofold. Firstly, I wanted to bring the huge problems faced daily by these very special children and their families, to the attention of the wider community. They face a lifelong commitment that for most of us would be unbearable; and often with inadequate services to give them the support they need. I have tried to include some examples and quotations from their lives that highlight the underlying ethical issues. Often, in the neonatal intensive care unit, decisions are made under extreme pressure, very quickly after delivery. Most parents desperately want their child to live, but should every very premature baby be resuscitated? Who should make such decisions? Are doctors the best people to decide, bearing in mind that it is the parents who will ultimately be responsible for the child if it is badly damaged?

Secondly, I feel strongly that the issues raised when very premature babies are saved do not affect only doctors and parents; they have much broader implications. Decisions made at this crucial stage of treatment indirectly affect us all. There are huge problems in the NHS and social services; most are to do with resources, staff shortages and under-funding. Government money allocated in one area cannot be spent elsewhere. As a society it is important that we understand where and how we order our priorities. I hope that this book helps to raise some awareness of the concerns I feel.

PART 1

The impact of prematurity on the child and family

Part 1 outlines the latest developments in neonatal intensive care, and explains how very premature babies can now be saved. It also describes the disabilities that such babies may suffer, and the impact on parents and families.

PART CONTENTS

2

The background and context of neonatal intensive care

> One of the most morally awesome and powerful aspects of perinatal care is the ability to affect a baby's very being. Never have their physical capabilities, their developmental capacities, their mental abilities, their genetic makeup, as well as their actual existence, been quite so much in the hands of health professionals.
>
> (Mitchell 1986, p. 342)

Despite major advances in treatments for premature babies, doctors still have not managed to stem the rising tide of premature births.

During the 1950s, the development of special care units for premature and low birth weight babies was initiated. Prior to that, as John Wyatt and Andrew Spencer (1992) point out, the only care available was to keep them warm and fed by mouth. Consequently, most would have died naturally in the first few hours or days of life, from complications arising from their prematurity.

In the early days, oxygen therapy was first introduced to counteract respiratory distress syndrome, but unfortunately many infants suffered retinal damage and subsequent blindness until the high concentrations of oxygen were discovered to be the cause.

Since then, there have been major improvements in techniques and equipment: the 1960s saw the introduction of nasogastric feeding and the beginnings of artificial ventilation. In the 1970s, methods of examining tiny samples of blood were discovered, facilitating the diagnosis of abnormalities, and umbilical catheterisation became a common procedure.

During the 1980s and 1990s these techniques have been developed, and more techniques have been discovered. Today babies of lower and lower birth weight and gestational age are being treated, because the technology for saving their lives is improving at such a rapid rate.

- Cranial ultrasound is used to reveal and monitor brain damage.
- Miniature cannulae are now being used for the intravenous treatment of the tiniest babies with fluids and antibiotics, and for regular blood transfusions needed to replace blood taken for tests.
- More sophisticated methods of mechanical ventilation are now available.
- Surfactant therapy involves the use of an artificial lung lubricant, to help inflate the immature lung tissue of the very premature baby.
- Transcutaneous monitoring of blood gases is possible.
- Jaundice may be treated with phototherapy.

In fact, as Pam Miller (1996, p. 123) points out, 'Equipment for measuring every conceivable parameter is constantly refined and most vital functions can now be sustained for some time at least, by some form of machinery'.

However, the very specialist knowledge, skills and technologies, which can interfere with the natural processes of life, bring with them profoundly complicated ethical dilemmas and, as R Mitchell (1986, p. 430) points out: 'The more one can do, the more one should consider whether one should do it'.

THE ROLE OF THE NEONATAL NURSE

The job of the neonatal nurse is extremely satisfying, but is also very demanding. Over the past decade the role has changed and developed, reflecting the new responsibilities brought by advances in technology. Today's neonatal nurse practitioners (NNP) have trained and qualified in the more advanced techniques of critical care and management of the newborn. According to Maggie Redshaw it was expected that as these specialised practitioners developed their skills and expertise, they would begin to become more involved in making decisions about patient care treatment and take on some of the responsibilities of their medical colleagues. So now the NNP undertakes a wide range of clinical procedures, which include:

- Inserting intravenous cannulae
- Ordering X-rays and infection screens
- Blood sampling
- Performing lumbar punctures
- Inserting chest drains.

They are also responsible for teaching other neonatal nurses, midwives and junior medical staff.

However, the role of the NNP differs from hospital to hospital. Depending on the size of the unit, they may work on a rota with junior medical staff; they may have responsibility for a few babies in intensive care; they may also take on technical tasks for the other infants in the unit.

The NNP uses her considerable clinical skills to care for babies; she also spends much time with distressed and often grieving parents. She usually knows each baby very well, understanding their responses to the way they are handled and fed especially if they have been on the unit for several weeks. However tiny the infants, they all seem to develop their own ways of reacting to the different stimuli in their little world.

The NNP is usually the first person with whom the parents have contact when they come onto the unit: they learn to trust her, and rely on her for information and support. She is a useful link between the parents and other professionals, especially when a multidisciplinary approach is required. As Miller (1996) observes, she may find that because of her unique situation in relation to the child, she has a greater understanding of what affect the treatment is having, on both baby and family. She may feel that ongoing aggressive therapy is causing more harm than good, or that the decision to withdraw treatment is made too quickly; sometimes, parental insistence that ventilation is continued, in the face of evidence that the child has suffered irreparable damage, is not easy to live with.

The neonatal nurse has a function in keeping the lines of communication open between parents and doctors. She becomes an advocate for the infant, while at the same time listening to parents and helping them to reach their own decisions, or helping them explain their views to other professionals. Sometimes she may find herself in conflict with doctors, or even with parents, if she cannot agree that the course they are following is in the baby's best interest. Since the baby cannot speak for itself, it is up to the nurse to decide when drugs are needed or whether the child is suffering if feeds are withdrawn. Sometimes she may be reluctant to administer pain-killing drugs that may shorten the baby's life, if she feels there is little evidence of the baby being distressed.

Miller (1996) stresses that, because the neonatal nurse will inevitably encounter these kinds of ethical dilemmas in her daily routines, it is important that she is clear about her own position regarding her beliefs and standpoint in relation to the tasks she may be asked to perform. An appreciation of ethical principles and legal guidelines will help give her the confidence to be more proactive in her role.

Open discussion, involving all parties, on the way treatment should proceed is essential, so that all those involved can work with integrity, in the belief that their views are being heard and seriously considered. In the end it is obviously the paediatrician who will make the ultimate decision, but the neonatal nurse's input to that decision is vitally relevant to the development of an appropriate care plan. Miller (1996) suggests that a combination of factors must be considered, including:

- the views of the neonatologist
- the severity of the defect
- availability of surgical treatment
- the gestational age of the infant
- parental attitude.

If active treatment is not considered advisable, the care plan should address all the infant's physical and emotional needs, along with those of the family. Miller (1996) maintains that if such a care plan is not implemented, we are conveying negative messages about the value of a severely damaged child's life.

When a baby dies, the neonatal nurse's role is essential to the way parents will remember their child. Sensitivity to their wishes is crucial; encouraging them to grieve in whatever way seems right for them, so that they may begin to come to terms with their loss and the possible feelings of guilt and remorse following a decision to withdraw treatment.

DEFINITION OF EXTREME PREMATURITY

Extreme prematurity can be defined as live birth at less than 28 completed weeks of gestation. (Wyatt and Spencer 1992, p. 5)

The length of a normal pregnancy is usually 40 weeks, or 279 days, and the gestational age of the foetus is calculated from the first day of the mother's last menstrual period. Any baby born before 37 weeks' gestation is considered to be premature, but most of those born close to full term generally do well, with few long-term problems. There are three categories of very premature babies:

- **moderate** prematurity is a birth between 35–37 weeks
- **very** premature births occur between 29–34 weeks
- **extreme** prematurity is a birth between 24–28 weeks.

The risk of complications grows as gestational age decreases. Today, with the aid of sophisticated technology, it is becoming possible to save more and more babies, even those born extremely prematurely. So babies born just over halfway through pregnancy are sometimes treated to keep them alive.

In strictly legal terms, a foetus that shows any signs of life following complete expulsion from the mother's body should be classified as a live birth. However, Wyatt and Spencer (1992) point out that the recorded incidence of premature births varies from region to region, because the precise definition of a live birth differs from hospital to hospital and even between individual labour wards. Some hospitals are known to record those foetuses described above as dead at birth; therefore they are categorised as a spontaneous abortion rather than a neonatal death. As a result they do not appear in the statistics for live births.

Jon Tyson (1995) points to the difficulty in accurately pinpointing the exact gestational age of a premature baby and emphasises the problems that a small margin of error can produce. If a woman's menstrual cycle is irregular or she has an uncertain menstrual history, making predictions about the estimated date of delivery can be very difficult, and it is difficult to categorise premature infants. Generally, babies born weighing less than 2500 grams (5lb 5oz) are considered premature, but sometimes premature babies can weigh more than that. Therefore, doctors use a combination of gestational age and birth weight to establish which infants can be designated as 'very premature'.

WHAT ARE THE CAUSES OF EXTREME PREMATURITY?

Despite major improvements in treatments for very premature babies, that the number of premature births has continued to rise, and the UK has one of the highest rates of premature birth in Europe. There is much speculation about the reasons for this. Often doctors just do not know what causes premature birth; there may be a number of contributory factors.

Maternal causes

- Today, the number of pregnancies among women over the age of thirty-five is increasing. Age alone may be a factor, but these women may also have pre-existing conditions like hypertension, stress, gynaecological infections, obesity and diabetes that put them in a higher risk category.
- Sommerfield (2001) cites a study by Dr Donald Mattison which found that black women are twice as likely to give birth prematurely as white women, although there are no obvious reasons for this.
- Pre-eclampsia is a potentially dangerous condition in which the mother's blood pressure is raised, causing fluid retention and proteinuria. The placental blood supply is interrupted, causing problems with the transfer of nutrients from mother to baby. If the condition does not respond to treatment, it is often necessary to induce an early labour.
- Placenta praevia is a condition in which the placenta is attached wholly or partly to the lower part of the uterus. It cannot stretch with the growing womb in later pregnancy and begins to detach, causing blood loss and early labour.
- Polyhydramnios, a condition where there is excessive fluid around the baby, causes the uterus to become overstretched, resulting in early onset of labour.
- Early rupture of the membranes may cause premature delivery.
- Previous history of premature delivery or threatened miscarriage can be a risk factor.
- Stress, either physical or mental, can be a risk factor.
- It is also thought that socio-economic factors may play a part: poor diet and general health are contributory factors.

Foetal causes

- One of the obvious causes, as Julia Sommerfield (2001) points out, is the increase in the number of multiple births. When there is more than one baby, labour is likely to be early, and the babies are likely to have low birth weights.
- Foetal abnormalities are another cause of premature birth.

CAN PREMATURITY BE PREVENTED?

It is not easy to predict the outcome when a very premature birth occurs, but it is generally accepted that gestational age is a much more important factor than birth weight in determining the prognosis of an extremely premature baby.

> The limit of viability is still considered to be 23–24 weeks' gestation, although survival at those ages can be considered more of a tragedy than a triumph.
>
> (Allen, Donahue and Dusman 1993)

The best remedy for prematurity is early detection and treatment of underlying causes such as pre-eclampsia. To reduce the risk of giving birth prematurely, doctors recommend that women take sensible measures in pregnancy by having regular antenatal care, not smoking or taking recreational drugs or alcohol, and immediately reporting any unusual symptoms which might indicate complications or signs of premature labour.

Research into the causes and prevention of premature birth is ongoing, some of the projects being sponsored by charities or funded by grants from the National Lottery.

One project reported by Cerebra, the charity helping brain injured children, at the University of Leeds, is examining possible links to the triggering of premature births. It is generally accepted that an infant born at 32 weeks' gestation or earlier is 40 times more likely to develop cerebral palsy; some think that the cause could have a genetic link. The project is due to publish results in late 2002 on a study of 100 women, to evaluate a group of 50 who gave birth at full term without complications and another group of 50 who had premature births, to see how they compare.

Tommy's charity is at present funding a number of research projects, detailed on their website (see Appendix) which are concerned with understanding and preventing premature labour, and preventing health problems in small or preterm babies.

• One study is investigating the possible causes of early rupture of the membranes, one of the commonest reasons for premature birth. Membranes that have ruptured early show signs of changes in their structure, causing possible weakness. Researchers have identified the enzymes responsible and are currently investigating how they are produced and controlled; they hope that in time their work may lead to the development of drugs to counteract the problem.
• Certain proteins are also known to act within the cells of the membrane surrounding the amniotic fluid and research is currently in progress as to whether they play any significant role in the changes which lead to early rupture.
• Hormone activity is also being scrutinised; recent findings show that levels of oestriol in the saliva of pregnant women rise before both normal and premature birth. It is hoped that this could improve the ability to predict premature labour and to develop treatments to help prevent it.
• New studies are seeking to identify drugs that will delay labour and, importantly, carry no side effects for mother and baby.
• Research is looking into the causes of bacterial vaginosis, a condition present in many women who go into premature labour.
• Researchers are trying to establish whether certain hormones produced by the placenta (especially Activin A) are responsible for some of the symptoms of pre-eclampsia.
• Drugs which are used to help premature babies with breathing problems may also help infants during traumatic labour and delivery. researchers are looking for ways of using these drugs to aid cardiovascular efficiency during the birth of very premature babies, so that more blood is directed to the brain, helping to prevent brain damage. It is thought that injecting the drugs directly into the baby in the uterus, rather than via the mother's placenta, will improve their effectiveness.
• Studies into foetal brain development and activity, particularly within the regions controlling sight, hearing and foetal learning, are being undertaken in the hope of developing preventative treatments for cerebral palsy and problems of prematurity.
• The response of the liver and other organs to serious infection in preterm babies is being studied, in order to improve the care of infants with severe infections.

SOME COMPARATIVE STATISTICS

When studying the following statistics, it is important to realise that each hospital will have its own variation on these figures. What may be true in one intensive treatment unit will not necessarily hold true for another. Unfortunately, it is also now well known that in any branch of medicine, the treatment patients receive can differ depending on where they live.

Nevertheless, the following represent the general trends in the long-term view for the very premature baby.

Britain

In the United Kingdom approximately 650,000 babies are born every year and approximately one in four has some neurological problem. There are a number of possible reasons for this, one of which is prematurity. According to Sue Summers (2002) we have a worse record than most other European countries in the actual care of premature infants; at the same time, paradoxically, we are responsible for many new techniques and machines. The UK has the highest rate of premature births in Europe, and the second highest rate of infant mortality. She points to a report by the British Association of Perinatal Medicine, which says there is no guarantee that all sick babies will be treated in fully equipped units by properly trained staff.

According to Hadley (2000), 40,000 families per year are affected by premature births. Ten per cent of babies born before 37 weeks' gestation are classified as 'extremely premature' (less than 28 weeks gestation), weighing less than approximately 1000 grams (2lb 3oz). Approximately half of these babies will survive. In one sense neonatology is a victim of its own success; many more babies survive each year and more and more are being treated at earlier and earlier gestation.

According to Mitchell (1986), the survival rate for babies weighing between 500 and 700 grams (1lb 1oz–1lb 9oz) is around 30% and for gestations of 24–26 weeks, about 50%. But what of those who survive? Miller (1996) maintains that around 15% of survivors with birth weights below 1000 grams (2lb 3oz) have a 'significant handicap'. The increase in survival of very preterm babies during the 1980s was accompanied by a sharp increase in the rate of cerebral palsy in this group.

The frequency of cerebral palsy decreased with increasing gestational age and birth weight. Factors which seemed to be associated with increased risk of cerebral palsy after adjustment for gestational age were chorioanionitis, prolonged rupture of the membranes and maternal infection. Other causes may include respiratory and cardiovascular complications, bacterial infections, neonatal seizures, tube feeding and low sodium, with fits severely increasing the risk.

In August 2000, a study by EPIcure (Hadley p40) found that severe disability was common among babies born extremely early. All the children in the study were born at less than 25 weeks' gestation between March and December 1995 in the UK and Ireland. During that time 811 children were born, and 497 died in hospital. 300 were evaluated at age 30 months. The researchers found that:

- 19% had severe delayed development
- 11% had below average development
- 28% had severe neuromotor disability
- 138 children (just under 50% of survivors) had disabilities like blindness and cerebral palsy
- 64 children were severely disabled.

According to Hadley, other research in 1995 concluded that babies weighing less than 750 grams (1lb 10oz) at birth had lower cognitive ability, psychomotor skills and academic achievement, poor social skills and behavioural problems.

Hadley points out that these are average figures and may not accurately reflect results in 'state of the art' neonatal intensive care units. Nevertheless they are depressing results: for however successful their initial treatment, the odds will always be stacked against these children.

America

According to Woodrum (1998) in an American study, those babies born before 25 weeks' gestation, along with those born with severe congenital abnormalities, have 100% mortality without aggressive intervention. A long-term follow up of those very low birth weight babies who survived intensive care showed that while most are normal, a significant number were left with either minor or major disabilities.

A 1993 study of babies born at 22-25 weeks, by MC Allen, PK Donoghue and AE Dusman, published in the *New England Journal of Medicine,* was stated that none lived who was born before 23 weeks. Of those born at 23 weeks 83% had severe brain damage, as did 64% of those born at 24 weeks. By 25 weeks gestation the number fell sharply to 13%.

Margaret Sykes quotes from Williams Obstetrics (1997), describing several studies looking at outcomes for very premature babies born during the 1980s, when more aggressive treatments began to be undertaken. After two years none survived who had been born at 23 weeks' gestation. Of those who survived birth at 24 weeks, only 6% did not have severe health problems, but 50% of those born at 25–26 weeks were found to be doing well.

Another study, undertaken by Hack in Ohio between 1992 and 1995, observed the longer term outcomes of babies with extremely low birth weights who were admitted to intensive care, but had no other major congenital malformations. Of 333 babies born weighing below 1000 grams (2lb 3oz), 241 survived to 20 months of age. The researchers assessed 221 children of these remaining children, whose average gestational age was 26.4 weeks, for cognitive and neurosensory development. Results showed that 54 children (24%) had major neurosensory abnormalities. and 92 children (42%) had a subnormal cognitive development. It was also found that children who survive very premature birth have a much greater risk of sudden infant death syndrome.

WHAT DOES IT ALL MEAN? A SUMMARY

Predicting outcomes for very premature babies immediately following birth is a very imprecise science. If a baby survives birth at 23-24 weeks' gestation there is evidence to suggest that they will have at least some degree of disability. Brain injury and cerebral palsy are the most significant problems and at this point in gestation there appears to be an equal chance of four outcomes, although there will be some babies within each group who do not exactly fit every criteria.

- **Group 1**: Children with no disabilities. They operate within the normal spectrum of intelligence and physical abilities, but may be small for their age or have some slight visual problems causing them to wear glasses.

- **Group 2**: These children will suffer mild handicaps, with intelligence slightly below normal. In school they may be affected by attention deficit, emotion problems or hyperactivity. They are sometimes clumsy but can generally manage normal physical performance. Some will have learning disabilities, difficulty with language and social skills that could entail special educational needs.
- **Group 3**: In this category one would expect to find children falling below the normal range of intelligence. They will be slow in reaching their developmental milestones and will probably suffering some degree of cerebral palsy, causing awkwardness in walking or fine motor problems (such as reaching and grasping) which will require ongoing physiotherapy. They could be visually impaired and many of them will never be able to lead an independent existence.
- **Group 4**: These children are severely disabled and could have profound and multiple learning disabilities. They suffer from severe cerebral palsy that affects sight, hearing, gross and fine motor movements. They will be totally dependent on others for most of their everyday needs. Almost all of these children will be educated in a special school environment.

3

The very premature baby: a profile

CHARACTERISTICS OF A VERY PREMATURE BABY

According to Betty Sweet (1984) there are two categories of low birth weight infants:

1. Preterm babies born between 24 and 37 weeks, gestation.
2. 'Light for dates' babies. Due to intrauterine malnutrition, these infants fall into the tenth percentile for their gestational age.

Some babies fall into both categories, but in this context we shall be concentrating on those with very low birth weight who need intensive and sometimes aggressive medical interventions to save or prolong their lives. They often weigh less than 1000 grams and have very immature natural life support systems.

In order to ascertain any newborn baby's condition immediately after birth the midwife uses a method of assessment called the Apgar score. This is done by observing five vital signs and awarding a score of 0, 1 or 2 to each of the following:

- Heart rate
- Respiratory effort
- Muscle tone
- Reflex irritability
- Colour.

These observations are repeated every five minutes until a score of between eight and ten is achieved. However, if a very low Apgar score (less than 3) is recorded in those first few minutes, this indicates the need for immediate resuscitation. Obviously, the more premature the infant, the more immature are all his vital functions. Lungs, heart, brain, liver and intestinal tract are now forced to operate independently from the uterus, and if the baby is very premature these organs may not yet be mature enough to function effectively. A thorough assessment of the situation is completed within the first few hours to investigate the condition of all these organs, and an ultrasound scan of the cranium and nervous system may be carried out.

Immediately after birth, the very premature baby is usually inactive and has little subcutaneous fat: prominent surface veins show through the wrinkled red skin of his abdomen and chest. Body temperature is difficult to maintain because of the immature neurological system that controls body heat, so the infant is dried off, placed in a warm blanket, and then nursed in a humidified incubator or under a radiant heater. The tiniest of these very premature infants will probably only have 40–50mls of blood in circulation, so regular blood transfusions are needed to replace samples taken to monitor blood gases or other potential complications, although it is possible to use transcutaneous methods for some of the tests.

The suck and swallow reflex will probably not develop for a number of weeks, so tube feeding is required and intravenous lines are established so that fluids, nutrients and antibiotics can be administered.

Characteristically, a very low birth weight baby has a large soft head, with wide sutures and fontanelles, which seems out of proportion to the rest of the body. The abdomen appears swollen and the chest small. Lunago or silky hair may cover the head and trunk, and nails and ears are soft, the latter having no cartilage. Boy infants may have undescended testicles and in girls the labia minora is not covered by the labia majora.

The infant needs a quiet, noise-free environment in which to thrive. Stimulation is kept to a minimum; even loud conversations can cause signs of stress such as frowning, yawning, sneezing, hiccups, or a change in heart rate or colour.

Most will remain in hospital until their estimated date of delivery draws near; an infant born at 23 weeks would be expected to stay for a further 17 weeks. The stay in the neonatal intensive care unit varies depending on their gestational age and maturity, and how well they progress. When they are no longer considered to be in danger, they are transferred back to the unit or nursery for care until discharge from hospital.

POTENTIAL HEALTH RISKS FOR THE VERY PREMATURE BABY

Prematurity is one of the major causes of serious illness in newborn babies. Because they find it difficult to adapt to extrauterine life, these infants are prone to further complications that could affect their future health and survival, depending on the gestational age and maturity.

- **Mental retardation**: Prematurity is not necessarily a major cause of mental retardation, but extremely premature babies are more prone to it than full term healthy babies. A number of the following conditions increase the risk.
- **Birth asphyxia and apnoea**: Very premature babies have problems breathing because of the immaturity of their lungs. An Apgar score of 4–7 records moderate asphyxia; a score below that indicates an urgent situation requiring immediate intervention. Most extremely premature infants require artificial ventilation from the beginning.
- **Respiratory Distress Syndrome (RDS)**: All babies born before 35 weeks' gestation are at risk. There is insufficient surfactant in the lungs, causing incomplete expansion of the alveoli during inhalation, so many of the tiny sacs collapse and never recover. Surfactant is the fatty substance in mature lungs, which helps to keep them expanded. One of the major advances in treatment for this condition in recent years has been the introduction of surfactant therapy, which has been a key contributor to saving life. With this treatment many more infants begin to slowly improve, so that eventually they can be weaned off respiratory support until they are breathing independently. In addition, a steroid, betamethasone, may be injected into the mother before delivery; this aids in the maturation of the baby's lungs and helps to produce surfactant.

Unfortunately, not all treatments for RDS are so helpful. It has been discovered that the drug dexamethasone, which has been used to counteract the condition and to prevent chronic lung disease in premature babies, is associated with increased risks of cerebral palsy and developmental delay. In a long-term study,

159 children were assessed for neurodevelopmental outcomes at 4 years of age. Some had been treated with the drug at birth; others were given a placebo. Findings showed that 55% of the treated children and 29% of the placebo group suffered developmental delay. Also, 49% of the treated children had cerebral palsy, even though 11 of them had normal ultrasound scans as neonates, as against 15% of the placebo group (Shinwell 2000).

Unfortunately for some babies, their lungs have suffered too much initial damage or are too immature, and death is inevitable.

- **Jaundice**: A lack of enzymes in the immature liver can lead to a dangerous rise in bilirubin, the product formed by the breakdown of red blood cells. Bilirubin can be deposited in the skin causing jaundice in babies. If the child is healthy and full term, this clears up naturally in a few days, but very premature babies may develop kernicterus, which can give rise to serious brain damage. Phototherapy is used to treat this problem.
- **Hypoglycaemia**: Very low levels of blood glucose may cause convulsions, lethargy, irritability, hypotonia, RDS apnoeic attacks, hypothermia, hunger and poor feeding.
- **Hypocalcaemia**: Low calcium levels can lead to twitching, tetany and convulsions; again, causing brain damage.
- **Neonatal infection**: Infections are quite common and premature babies are very susceptible to them. Any infection in very premature babies is potentially harmful because of the imminent threat of convulsions leading to permanent brain damage or death.
- **Retinopathy of prematurity**: This is common mainly in babies born earlier than 28 weeks' gestation. The blood vessels in the retina develop abnormally, and may cause the inner lining of the retina to detach from the outer lining. This is because their growth is not normally completed until a few weeks before birth and so full development has been interrupted.
- **Ventilation**: Although artificial ventilation saves the lives of thousands of premature babies every year, its use is not without risks. The very technology used to help babies breathe and keep them alive can also damage the lungs. This damage may lead to breathing problems in early childhood, even pneumonia, which may continue in some instances into adulthood.
- **Permanent residual scarring**: One problem that is not always considered until later in the child's life, and can be completely

overlooked by anyone who does not live with the issue, is the scarring left by some procedures in neonatal intensive care. Naturally, in the initial stages of deciding the course of treatment when an infant's life is at risk, this is something that is not even a subject for consideration. However, many parents, like Allison Martin (2001), have pointed out the effect that visible scars may have as the child grows into adulthood. While some scarring may fade with time, in other cases it can become bigger and create problems in adolescence. Unusual shaped or non-existent navels, or large abdominal or chest and back scars may become a considerable cause of embarrassment, particularly for a teenage girl, with today's fashions of bare midriffs and bikini swimwear. Some parents have reported more serious side effects, such as misinterpretation by strangers of scars on the wrists of some youngsters who had suffered cardiac arrests; they have sometimes been taken as evidence of attempted suicide. Scars around the neck and head area can affect hair growth, leaving little bald patches that are impossible to hide. In serious cases of scarring, plastic surgery may be the answer.

Many of the above potential problems caused by the immaturity of tiny organs can be overcome by fluids and drugs, because of their capacity for regeneration and new growth given time. Nevertheless, it has to be said that predicting the outcome for individual babies is still very difficult because of the number of uncertainties and exceptions surrounding their care. The main danger for the very premature infant is from trauma to the brain and central nervous system that has permanent and irreversible effects.

BRAIN INJURY AND ITS IMPLICATIONS

The main cause of brain injury in the very premature baby is severe bleeding in the brain. The tiny blood vessels inside the skull are underdeveloped and very fragile. They can burst very easily, causing extensive and possibly life-threatening trauma to the brain. The more premature the baby, the more risk there is of intraventricular haemorrhage (IVH), which is the most common form of brain bleed and is one indicator that will predict probable handicaps fairly well. Premature babies less than 34 weeks' gestation usually have a series of head ultrasounds during the first few days of life to monitor and detect these potentially fatal conditions. If a baby can escape the shock of a brain haemorrhage in the first three days of life they have passed a major obstacle.

Wyatt and Spencer (1992) name two major causes of brain injury in the very premature baby:

1. **Periventricular haemorrhage**: Minor degrees of cerebral haemorrhage are fairly frequent, but will have little or no effect on the baby. They are not associated with significant brain injury or long-term disability. Unilateral major bleeds into the parenchyma, the solid tissue in the brain, usually result in permanent brain injury and cerebral palsy leading to long-term disability. Major *bilateral* bleeds into the same area usually have far graver results, leading to severe brain injury and death. Bleeds of this kind almost always happens in the first few days after birth. If the child survives, there is an increased chance that they may develop hydrocephalus and/or complications arising from cerebral palsy, with the prospect of further ongoing surgery in the future.
2. **Hypoxic-ischaemic injury**: This is the most common cause of severe brain injury in survivors of premature birth. Sadly, it is not easy to detect in the early weeks, as it does not always show up on ultrasound, so the problem may not be detected for a while, sometimes not until after the child has left the special care unit.

In general, it is much easier to predict the outcome of a severe cerebral haemorrhage in the premature baby, for in these cases the child will almost always be severely disabled. However, here again a cautionary note is sounded; some may escape relatively unscathed and suffer only minor disabilities, while some babies with no bleeding to the brain will develop handicaps later.

CEREBRAL PALSY

Cerebral palsy is an umbrella term that covers a number of chronic disorders which result from an injury to the brain. The injury may have been caused by infection, accident or trauma at birth; it may have resulted from a congenital condition, or have no known cause.

In the UK alone about 1000 babies are born suffering from cerebral palsy each year, many of whom are very premature or of low birth weight. Babies born weighing less than 2500 grams (5$^{1}/_{2}$ lbs) or at less than 37 weeks' gestation, are at increased risk of cerebral palsy.

It is a neurological condition that may result in varying degrees of permanent physical and mental harm. The damage may be only slight, in which case the individual can lead a fairly normal life; however if the damage is more extensive symptoms may affect coordination of movement and speech, including shaking limbs, inability to sit unaided or to walk, problems with reaching and grasping, and loss of balance. It can also have a profound effect on the mental processes, leaving children with various degrees of learning disabilities that range from slight developmental delay and minor problems with speech and language to profound and multiple learning disabilities. It is also common for children with severe cerebral palsy to have fits or seizures; some will have minor attacks several times a day or week, others can be subject to quite major episodes.

4

The child and its family

THE EFFECTS OF PREMATURITY ON THE CHILD

In this section I would like to start with two case studies. Both children were very premature babies and suffered similar initial setbacks in the neonatal period. Their lives were saved by the skill and technology within the neonatal intensive care unit.

Kate was born at 25 weeks' gestation, by caesarean, weighing 750 grams (1lb 11oz). She is the first child of loving and fairly affluent parents.

During the first 24 hours she suffered breathing problems and needed to be resuscitated; these continued over the next few days in addition to which she suffered internal bleeding and needed a transfusion. She underwent physiotherapy on her tiny chest and tolerated a feed of $^{1}/2$ml breast milk every two hours via a nasogastric tube.

On the tenth day she suffered yet another setback. She developed a chest infection so antibiotics were prescribed and she was put back onto the ventilator. During the next few days she had several episodes when she stopped breathing and had to be resuscitated.

When Kate was nearly three weeks old, her parents were informed that she was to be transferred to a specialist children's hospital to undergo surgery for a hole in the heart as soon as a bed became available. At this point she was tolerating 5mls of breast milk every hour. Two days later they were still waiting for a theatre slot to become vacant. She was operated on at just three weeks old and returned to her original hospital later the same day, still on the ventilator and sedated with morphine. Two days later the morphine was discontinued and Kate began her feeding regime once more.

One week later she was reported to be doing well off the ventilator and on the CPAP (Continuous Positive Airway Pressure) machine. She was taking 7mls of milk every hour and had been out of the incubator for a cuddle with Mum.

At five weeks (30 weeks gestational age) she weighed 1100 grams (2lb 9oz) and could be taken off the CPAP machine for short spells. The CPAP applies air pressure to keep the tiny lungs expanded, via an endotracheal tube or via the nose. Her parents were delighted with the progress and were able to nurse her regularly on their visits to the special care unit.

Kate came out of intensive care after eight weeks and was transferred to the high dependency unit, weighing 1650 grams (3lb 10oz). She was being fed every three hours with 40mls milk and when sucking became too much for her, the nasogastric tube was reintroduced. At this point she could manage some short spells of breathing without the CPAP machine.

At the age of 13 weeks, and weighing 2500 grams $5^{1}/2$ lbs, she was discharged from hospital into the care of her parents. Kate is still too young for any potential learning disabilities to be assessed accurately. All the signs so far are encouraging, but it will not be known for some months, years even, whether she has been physically or mentally damaged by her premature delivery and treatment during the first few months of life.

Jennie lives with her mother and older brother in a second storey council flat in a big city complex. Her mother is young and finds it difficult to cope with the child's profound physical and mental needs alongside the demands of her other child, who is under school age. She often misses vital meetings with social workers and hospital appointments unless she is picked up and taken. Jennie has been hospitalised twice because of injuries and accidents around the home. Despite her many problems, she is a delightful child and a great favourite in school, with her ready smile and placid disposition.

Jennie began school aged two (special education begins early). She had suffered neurological damage after being ventilated after her birth at 25 weeks' gestation. She later developed hydrocephalus, has cerebral palsy with severe mental impairment and is profoundly deaf.

The cerebral palsy has affected all her limbs. Consequently she will never walk, sits only with the aid of special equipment, has great difficulty grasping and holding objects in her hands and needs to wear hearing aids in both ears in order that she may, hopefully, one day learn some language skills. However, because of her age and mental disability it was a constant battle to get her to wear them and keep them in.

In order for her to begin any learning process, Jennie needs specialist equipment:

- A standing frame so that she can see the world from an upright position when necessary.
- A chair, tailor-made for her specific measurements, which supports her head, shoulders, hips, knees and feet.
- A special buggy/wheelchair to support her when she is taken outside.
- Specialist play and learning equipment designed for children with multiple learning disabilities.

In addition, she has physiotherapy every day, to keep her limbs as mobile as possible. Jennie has spent many months in and out of hospital, needing treatment for a blocked shunt, intestinal blockage, breathing problems and minor accidents. These are in addition to routine visits to the hearing clinics and milestone checks.

Both these cases illustrate the effects of prematurity on an infant immediately after birth and the potential difficulties both the child and family will face after leaving hospital.

Obviously, many babies escape unscathed, as we hope that Kate may have done; others may suffer only minor neurological damage, but there are a growing number of children who are not so lucky. Damage may not always be so severe or have the same effect as Jennie's; nevertheless, most will have some degree of disability. For these children, development will always have to be carefully monitored and provision made for their special needs.

The growing child and its needs

In 1939, Dr Mary Shirley published her observations of the developmental characteristics of premature babies whose birth weight was less than 2300 grams (5lb). The children were examined between the ages of 6 months and 30 months (Helen Harrison 2002). Her findings included the following results:

- **Sensory acuity**: The premature child is more sensitive in auditory responses; they are more keenly aware of noise and more easily distracted by sounds than their full term counterparts. Visually, the child is attracted by bright colours and will focus on one particular object, sometimes ignoring other objects used to attract their attention.
- **Language development**: Some developmental delay will probably be experienced. Baby talk may persist longer than with full term infants.
- **Attention span**: In the toddler it is extremely short; they are easily distracted and activities need to be changed every few minutes. They find it very difficult to keep on task, except when they are working on motor skills. Paradoxically, here they will stay focused and working hard until they have to give up through sheer exhaustion. Often this results in a frustrated temper tantrum.

- **Manual motor control**: Difficulties with fine motor movements of the fingers can result in delays in developing pincer movements for grasping and reaching. Arm movements can be jerky and clumsy, causing them to overreach for objects, or spill and scatter toys. One unusual finding was that many premature babies were predominantly left-handed.
- **Gross motor development**: The premature baby will learn to sit up, crawl and walk later than the full term infant. Some, of course, may never reach one or all of those stages. Others may have some motor problems like poor posture or difficulty with walking and sitting.
- **Emotional development**: Generally, they seem to be more susceptible to stimuli than full term children; they can be shyer or more prone to outbursts of temper or frustration. On the one hand they can become hyperactive, and difficult to control, on the other hand they may be floppy, sluggish and deliberate in movements. Boys were more prone to temper tantrums than girls, while girls displayed more passive resistance and stubbornness.

Although these findings were published over 60 years ago, I find it fascinating that they are still relevant today. My own daily experience in the classroom with children like these (a lot of them far more disabled), bears out the accuracy of many of the characteristics Dr Shirley describes.

THE EFFECTS OF PREMATURITY ON THE FAMILY

> During the early years, we as mothers, all spent much time with our children, trying to make them appear normal. Most of us had not been told that they were mentally handicapped and we were left to discover this over a period of years. When the realisation finally came, we tended to avoid anything and anyone to do with mental handicap and had tremendous difficulty in accepting the inevitable.
>
> (MacLachlan et al 1989, p. 25)

This passage was written in 1989 by a group of mothers whose babies had been born in the early 1960s with severe mental and physical disabilities. The group came into being as a result of an appeal from social services for help from parents of young adults with severe learning disabilities. The extract shows the way these parents and children were treated forty years ago when their babies were born. No one gave them any indication that there might be something wrong; they were left to find out for themselves as time went on.

This illustration reminds me of the story of another young woman who gave birth to her first baby, a boy with Down's Syndrome, during that same decade. Even though the child had the obvious features of a Down's baby and other characteristics, neither the doctors in hospital, the district nurse or the GP said anything to the mother at all about her baby's condition. A veil of silence was drawn within the family circle; no one discussed it openly and everyone pretended that everything was fine. Although there was lots of support within the family, no one ever mentioned the fact that the little boy had Down's Syndrome until it was time for him to start school.

We have moved on somewhat in the forty years or so since then; doctors and nurses in neonatal intensive care units are now much more supportive and open about the condition and prognosis of very ill or damaged babies. Nevertheless, the birth of a very premature baby is still a devastating start for any family, and caring for the child can be an exhausting, frustrating and frightening experience. Many families feel completely unprepared for the struggles they face when they finally bring their infant home, and in a lot of cases their problems are only just beginning. Although the critical weeks in intensive care are now over, the effects of prematurity may impinge on their lives for many months or years to come; sometimes even, for the rest of their lives. Apart from the day-to-day routines in the care of any new baby, the parents of the very premature infant need to be aware of possible complications that might arise, and any resources that could help them cope better.

According to Mutch (1997), the traditional view of the family is no longer relevant. This has real implications for those caring for children with profound and multiple disabilities. The conventional notion of the stable married couple maintaining a caring home environment for their child forever cannot now be taken for granted. Divorce, single parents, cohabitation and mothers in full time employment have changed the whole concept of family life.

Psychological and emotional factors

Many parents describe their initial reactions to the discovery that one's child is severely disabled as shock, disbelief, anger, bitterness, confusion and guilt. These feelings can sometimes result in varying degrees of depression that may require treatment. The impact is devastating: what should have been a joyous experience, is turned to grief as the anticipation of bringing home a full term, healthy infant is lost.

The mother often feels extremely guilty. Even when she took great care during her pregnancy, she often questions whether it could be 'her fault' and agonises about whether she could have done anything to prevent it. She is left with no sense of satisfaction or relief after giving birth. For both parents it can be a blow to their dignity, self-esteem and self-confidence, leaving them with a sense of shame and responsibility for bringing the child into the world. Sometimes they can even begin to blame each other.

These are overwhelming feelings and engender extreme emotions, but it is important to understand that these are normal reactions, and are similar to the grieving process in bereavement. In fact, the shock can sometimes trigger a profound psychological threat and it is said that some parents experience something similar to the post-traumatic stress syndrome seen in people who have undergone or witnessed an extremely stressful incident.

The first hurdle for many parents is the shock of seeing their tiny infant for the first time in the neonatal intensive care unit. It is hardly possible to recognise the tiny human being amid all the wires and tubes attaching him or her to machines. Parents often have an overwhelming sense of helplessness and uselessness in the face of such technology. In the initial few days after birth it may be difficult for them to begin the bonding process with their child because of the practical problems of touching and holding them.

Even when things have gone well and the baby has made enough progress to be discharged, bringing them home may seem a terrifyingly daunting prospect. Parents who have been fully informed about their child's prognosis will have fears about how they will cope and what the future holds. Certainly difficult and challenging modifications will have to be faced in their way of life. Much greater parenting skills are needed, as the demands of the new baby have to be balanced against the needs of the rest of the household; and often the feedback from the child can be slow or even non-existent. One mother described the job of caring for her disabled son as mentally and physically hard work; she said that the whole family needs time to recharge their batteries:

It's very hard to admit it, but carers are human too.

(Claire McCarthy, Guardian Society 24.04.02, p. 9)

In the normal situation, however exhausted parents may feel when caring for a new baby, they are frequently rewarded for their efforts as they watch their child's progress, from the first smile, reaching for a toy, to sitting, crawling and walking. Parents with a physically and mentally disabled child have to put in far more effort and wait much longer to see the fruits of their work. It can be both frustrating and disheartening; however, the pleasure and satisfaction of a tiny breakthrough in their child's development is cause for much celebration.

Another mother very movingly described the feeling of fear, panic, powerlessness and numbness which grew as her child's disability became more conspicuous and the outlook became bleaker.

The shunt that relieved the pressure inside Jody's head became blocked and then infected. Ordinary colds carried him to the brink of death. Even when he was healthy, he needed a lot of medical supervision. When I was not visiting hospitals and doctors, I was trying to soothe a miserable baby. Jody cried most of the time, the anguished wail of a colicky infant. He rarely slept, and of course, we did not sleep either. I felt sorry for him and perhaps even sorrier for myself.

(Featherstone 1980, p. 5)

She further describes her parental fears that she will not be able to protect her child from what his future quality of life might be: increasing dependency on others for his most basic needs; the impact of being different, of discrimination or victimisation. But worst of all she fears what will become of him when she and her husband are too old to care for him. She feels that having a disabled child forces parents to view their advancing years with despair. There will never be any respite or freedom for them in the future, because their child can never be independent.

Others point to the fact that when their children were young, families whose children were 'normal' accepted them more easily, but as they grew older and became teenagers, then adults, it was far more difficult for them to gain acceptance from their more able peers.

When, as some parents fear, the time arrives when they can no longer care for their child at home, the normal feelings of pride and joy when youngsters leave home to go to university or to a new job are denied them. Often the domestic situation breaks down as parents grow older and their child has become a severely disabled adult; one parent may die or become ill, leaving the other with no option but to place their disabled son or daughter into residential care. Often preparation work has been done over many months or even years with professionals, to ease the transition for both the disabled person and the parents. Nevertheless, the move is never easy.

Instead of the positive feelings of a youngster 'leaving the nest', some parents may feel guilt, because they are abandoning him/her to other people's care, and anxiety about how their offspring will cope without them. The normal feeling of 'letting go' of one's children is intensified, because often, even when they have reached adult status, people with special needs are still thought of as children.

One 65-year-old mother described her feelings after she had been widowed and forced to consider putting her son with learning disabilities into residential care:

> Oh, my daughter agreed and my sister...They thought, yes, he should go. But you see, I resented that. Because he's MY child. There's part of you which says, who do they think they are? Would they do it to their own children?
>
> (Richardson 1989, p. 9)

Olshansky (1962, p. 190-193) points out that in normal circumstances of mourning, the bereaved have a chance of coming to terms with the loss of a loved one, but in this situation the child is still present, which makes it impossible for the parents to accept the fact that they will never see their offspring reaching the milestones of normal development. At each significant stage in the child's life, for example at the beginning and ending of their education, or when their peers are thinking of marriage or careers, their parents relive their original fears and anxieties for the future. He describes these feelings as 'chronic sorrow', continuous mourning for the loss of all hopes and expectations for that child.

Sometimes the unwitting attitude of friends and relatives can further add to parental stress. When they hear of the birth of a disabled child, they often feel unsure about how to approach or respond to the situation and are confused about whether to congratulate or console the new parents. These reactions can result in additional feelings of isolation and a sense of loneliness for the parents, in the face of their tragedy.

However, despite all that has been described above, it is difficult to predict the effect such a child will have on a family. While one family may be torn apart, not all families find it such a burden; for some the practice of living with and caring for a severely disabled child can be deeply moving and life-enhancing. The child becomes a cherished member of the family and they claim that the experience helps their understanding of other people's problems and they become more sensitive to the needs of the other members of the family.

The same mother whose disabled son had recently left home to move into residential accommodation movingly describes her feelings as she comes to terms with life without him around the home.

> The debit side of a handicapped child is that you are really tied for life. But the credit side is that there is somebody who loves you and it's a lovely form of love. There's no ifs or buts about it. It's a pure love and its lovely, you know. So you lose all this. And it's very shattering. It really is shattering.
>
> (Richardson 1989, p. 10)

Financial factors

There is no doubt that after the birth of a child with multiple and profound disabilities there are financial costs to be met. The impact may vary from family to family, but having a child with severe special needs imposes heavy strains on the family budget and the burden increases with the age of the child.

Mutch (1997) cites the studies of Quine and Pahl (1985) and Sloper and Turner (1993) that indicate that the parenting of a disabled child involves what she describes as a 'cycle of adversity'. The demands of caring may lead to the father (in a two parent family) having to take time off work, while the mother finds it difficult to get paid employment. This leads to financial problems and possible social isolation. The problems worsen as their income lessens, while their expenses increase as they face the costs of special equipment, clothing, adaptations, diet and heating bills. Even the family car needs to be bigger (and therefore more expensive) in order to accommodate a wheelchair and any other equipment that may be essential.

Other surveys have supported these findings. For example, Beresford (1995) surveyed 1300 families caring for children with severe learning disabilities and found that:

- 90% of lone parents relied on benefits
- 30% of two parent families relied entirely on benefits
- 75% reported 'going without'
- 40% described their housing as unsuitable for the child
- less than 25% of parents thought that all the needs of the child were being met.

In addition they have to cope with loss of sleep, and the exhaustion and physical strain of lifting, feeding, handling, toileting and bathing or changing an incontinent and steadily growing youngster. Often too, as time goes by, the child may begin to develop very demanding or challenging behaviours, making the parents' lives even more difficult.

For two parent families, where the husband is the main breadwinner, some have found their chances of promotion blocked, mainly because the family is less able to become mobile and move to other areas due to the demands of setting up new support systems in a strange area for their child.

Effects on siblings

> The needs of brothers and sisters should not be overlooked and they should be provided for as part of a package of services for the child with a disability.
>
> (Department of Health Guidance and Regulations 1991, para 6.4)

This statement appears to acknowledge that the presence of a disabled brother or sister will certainly have a dramatic impact on the lives of any other children within the family and according to Atkinson and Crawforth (1995), 80% of children with disabilities in 1989 had siblings who did not have disabilities.

It is well documented that the demands of caring for a very severely disabled youngster must inevitably affect the time and energy parents have to devote to their other children. This in turn may result in feelings of resentment and guilt on the part of the 'normal' offspring towards both their parents and the disabled brother or sister.

Sone (1995), in a National Children's Home survey, found that although many children helped care for, and loved, their disabled brother or sister, seven out of ten reported that they had been either bullied or teased at school because of their sibling's handicap. The same survey stressed that 98% of disabled children live at home, but in many instances the needs of the siblings were overlooked and they avoided talking to parents about their feelings.

One child who recognised his parents' stress commented:

> I find it hard to say things, because they are going through a lot of pressure right now, without making it even worse.
>
> (Newson and Davies 1994)

It is easy to see how resentfulness and jealousy can build up in these situations, if children regard themselves as being treated unfairly, especially when they find it difficult to build up a normal sibling relationship. Many youngsters in these circumstances, see themselves as miniature parents, taking on responsibilities for the disabled child, which can weigh heavily on young shoulders.

One mother described such a situation:

> We are his carers – we being his mum and dad and his brother and sister, who have also become carers without even realising it (one of my two children is only two and a half).
>
> (Claire McCarthy, Guardian Society 24.04.02, p. 9)

However, despite all the possibilities for negative effects on other children in the family, there is no consistent pattern. Families vary: all react in different ways, and the degree of disability can have a tremendous impact on how they cope. Therefore, it is far from clear how children are actually affected by having a very disabled brother or sister.

Tritt and Esses (1998) discovered that there can actually be beneficial effects, for some siblings of disabled children display a much more mature and caring outlook than many others in their age group; and an American study by Simeonsson and Bailey (1986) concluded that although there was a wide difference in sibling reaction to the same handicapping condition, older siblings, even those who were quite young themselves, who took on the role of teacher or trainer for their younger brother or sister, not only improved the development of the disabled child, but also enhanced their own personal competence and image. However, the same study found that younger or closer age siblings have much more difficulty in adjusting.

Effects on marriage or partnerships

Again, there are mixed findings from studies into whether caring for a disabled child is a factor in the breakdown of relationships or marriage. As Mutch pointed out (1997), traditional views of what family life is about are no longer true, so problems can be compounded when one partner is the natural parent and the other is the step parent.

The accumulation of different stressors can have a serious effect on their lives and relationship. The amount of time spent caring for the child can mean that time for oneself, each other and other members of the family is very limited, putting a further strain on relationships. Child-minding facilities are not cheap, particularly for a child with severe disabilities.

According to Quine and Pahl (1985) a child can act as a last straw to a failing relationship, or it can unite and improve it. As the parents of any child know, nothing prepares you for the demands and responsibilities of parenthood. It is exhausting enough when the child is healthy and reaching the normal developmental milestones without problems. When the child is multiply disabled, life is much more difficult. Even the strongest relationships need to be supported sometimes, but if the bond is weak, then the prospect of bringing up a child with severe learning disabilities can be too much, especially when the parents are relatively young.

Cooke and Bradshaw (1986) and Sabbeth and Leventhal (1984) have concluded that, because it is difficult to assess what the state of any relationship was before the child was born, no clear findings emerge.

However, one surprising conclusion came from another survey by Byrne, Cunningham and Sloper (1988): it was that the presence of a partner is likely to alleviate stress, even if that partner is perceived not to be very supportive.

From this, one can assume that any partner is better than no partner in a family with special needs (however, personally I would have thought that in many cases it could have exactly the opposite effect). Nevertheless it has been shown that it is single parents, mainly, of course mothers, who experience the highest levels of stress. Byrne et al suggest the possible explanation that two parent families are more likely to receive more physical and financial support than someone on their own.

WHAT ARE THE ONGOING SERVICES NEEDED BY THE FAMILY FOR THE LIFETIME OF THEIR SEVERELY DISABLED CHILD?

Medical: The Health Service

From the moment of delivery, the very premature baby will spend the next few weeks, even months, in the neonatal intensive care unit. After discharge from hospital there is the prospect of regular hospital check ups, with the possibility of further major surgical interventions. Alongside this there will be ongoing input from the local GP and health visitor. As the child grows, he/she will probably need regular physiotherapy, occupational therapy and, if behavioural problems arise, the expertise of child psychiatrists. Of course, not all children require all of these health service resources, but in my experience as a teacher of children with profound learning disabilities, a high percentage do require most of them at some point in their lives.

Paediatric care is usually ongoing in the early years but parents or carers often need to request a medical check up for an older person with disabilities, rather than it being a routine procedure.

Housing needs

Even if families are able to stay in their present home, all will need help to adapt their present living space to accommodate any special equipment. Ramps, door widening, bathroom hoists, lifts for moving up and down stairs, or downstairs bedrooms and toilets will be necessary as the child gets older.

Social Services provision

The Chronically Sick and Disabled Persons' Act 1970 authorises the local authority to make an assessment of the child's needs, and the Children Act 1989 (Section 17) specifies a unified approach to services for disabled people. It urges the Social Services department to work with Education and Health and the voluntary sector to aim for 'lives which are as normal as possible' for their clients. Many of the parents (particularly the lone parent) would not be able to cope without the support of a social worker.

As well as being counsellors, they help organise respite care, special holidays, play schemes, and support in mainstream nurseries or playgroups, so that parents may have some time for themselves and their other children. The service is ongoing and the aim is to achieve a continuity of care so that however disabled the client, as they get older they are helped to achieve as much autonomy as possible when making choices about their lives. In some cases an advocate can be appointed, who represents the person at case conferences or whenever their future is being considered. The idea is to appoint someone who has no vested interest in whatever choices are being made and can therefore listen objectively and help everybody reach a decision, which is truly in the best interest of the client. Some might question the implications this might have for parental autonomy; if they are still the major carers for their offspring, should they also have the right to decide what is in their best interest? Certainly the role of advocate needs to be handled with great sensitivity: the opinions of everyone should be weighed very carefully, not least the parents, whose responsibilities go on from year to year, long after the professionals have moved on.

Education

The education of children with severe learning disabilities has seen major advances over the past few decades. Today, the child with special needs has a statutory right to education from the age of two years up to the age of nineteen. The statement of his needs is laid down in law and he is assessed according to that need. At present, all children with profound and multiple disabilities are educated within a special school setting, but the policy is for all children to be integrated as far as possible with their peer group. So, many with less severe needs are being educated in mainstream establishments with trained staff to support them.

Special schools have a very high pupil/teacher ratio. The staff are more highly paid than mainstream teachers, making the service extremely expensive. In my own class of six children with profound and multiple learning problems, we had one teacher and two specially trained classroom assistants. The teaching methods for children with profound and multiple learning difficulties are based on a sensory/motor approach designed to give them appropriate experiences to teach them about the world around them. The curriculum is based on the belief that however profoundly disabled a pupil may be, they should be given the opportunity to develop whatever potential they may have and learn some degree of autonomy and choice in life.

The physiotherapist played a major role in my school, spending time with individual pupils and teaching staff correct ways of positioning, handling and lifting pupils with multiple physical disabilities. This was important not only so that staff did not injure themselves, but so that children were always as comfortable as possible while working or playing. In order for them to gain as much as possible from their experiences, every child had several large pieces of equipment to assist them with learning. Each piece was tailor-made to fit the individual: standing frames, enabling them to view the world from a vertical position, chairs designed to support the ankles, knees, hips, shoulders and neck which could be adapted so that the pupil could get maximum benefit from every classroom activity. We had specially-designed play equipment, for children with extreme physical disabilities; a jacuzzi in the classroom, a hydrotherapy pool and a multisensory room on site. Here they could experience water therapy, aromatherapy massage, and interactive programmes to stimulate all their senses, and begin to learn how to control their own environment.

Outside the classroom, we built a multisensory garden for them to enjoy.

For all these activities, we relied on extra staff to help. For every physical activity it was essential to work on a one-to-one basis, so all special schools rely heavily on volunteers and students, and fortunately most schools have a pool of people who give their time to this cause.

However, handling children with profound and multiple disabilities requires skill and expertise, so all those who volunteer have to be willing to learn these skills. Even midday assistants who help to feed those pupils who are unable to eat unaided need special training. Mouth and tongue movements, chewing and swallowing are not only used for digesting food, but can be vital in the process of learning to speak, so our speech therapists had a good deal of input during times when the children were eating and drinking. Snack times and lunch times were not only times of recreation but essential learning periods, when each child had a set programme to aid in their speech and language development. In addition there is input from educational psychologists, music and drama therapists who are often employed on a sessional basis which is extra to the main school budget. Many of these essential extra services are paid for by voluntary contributions and fund-raising events.

Conclusion

All the above-mentioned services work separately and jointly to give as much support and care to the family as possible. As we all know, services and expertise are both scarce and expensive, and there are often huge gaps between the reality and the ideal, raising many ethical issues surrounding the allocation of resources for these very special people and their families.

Some argue that it is wrong to fight to save the life of a baby who may grow up to be so badly damaged that the quality of life for them and their family is too much to bear. They suggest that treatment should be withheld from some very premature babies right from the start and they should be allowed to die in peace. By comparing the probable future quality of life of the infant against the social and economic costs to the family and society they feel that the burdens on family and society far outweigh any benefits to the child. They assert that the lives of parents and other siblings need to be considered too, for the lives of everyone will be changed and limited forever by the impact of caring for the multiply disabled child. The interests of the family as a whole have to be weighed against the needs of the disabled child and there is a limit to how much a family should be expected to stand.

Others challenge this view as too utilitarian, saying that the worth or value of a disabled child's life should not be viewed from the perspective of what its potential effect or role will be within the family. Robinson and Stalker (1993) believe that the basic assumption that the cost to the family and society outweighs the advantages for the child is false: these things cannot be measured. Even if these costs are extremely high, how can they be measured against the cost to the child: he/she has to sacrifice life itself. The infant's life is intrinsically valuable, irrespective of how it affects the lives of others, so the effects of neonatal treatment decisions on the family are considered to be irrelevant. Any deviation from this principle may lead to the slippery slope towards involuntary euthanasia and the concept that one's right to life depends solely on the utilitarian judgements about social worth.

The problem of who should decide on such a crucial issue is another source of debate. What happens if parents and doctors do not agree about the next stage of treatment? Some feel that parents are in the best position to decide about the future of their child; others say that doctors should make such crucial decisions because parents cannot always be relied upon to make rational decisions at such an emotional time.

All these ethical issues begin to emerge as we see the effects that prematurity has on the child and its family. As the issue of justice and allocation of resources for people with special needs is such an important issue, the final section of this book is dedicated to that subject.

5

Counselling and care: support for parents and staff

Most parents whose child spent time in a neonatal care unit have vivid memories of the period: the details stay with them forever. From parental accounts of their experiences, it is obvious that the quality and type of support they receive varies, not only from hospital to hospital, but also from individual to individual, within the profession. Some report a very high level of care, receiving compassionate, sensitive treatment; others have very different stories to tell, and they are left with lasting feelings of anger and frustration.

SUPPORT FOR PARENTS

Immediately after birth

The birth of a very premature baby is not a beginning that anyone would wish for, and parents experience a mixture of feelings. The important thing is for hospital staff to be sensitive to, and sufficiently trained to deal with, the wide range of responses that they may encounter.

Many hospitals are now well equipped to pass on the education and counselling skills required in the modern neonatal intensive care unit and most staff who choose to work on such a unit have a caring and empathetic approach to parents. Encouraging parents and reassuring them about the frightening array of tubes and needles with which they are presented should come as second nature. Unfortunately this is not always the case. Insufficient funding and resources for training leave some areas of neonatal practice sadly lacking in adequately trained staff to deal with the sensitive issues which surround prematurity, disability and death.

Parents and infants must be treated with respect. Parents need to feel that they are an important factor in the recovery of their baby by helping with its care, so that the bonding process can begin as soon as possible. They need to feel that they are part of the decision-making process and that they are being dealt with truthfully and compassionately. For this to happen, it is essential for parents to be kept informed and consulted about the different courses of treatment or tests; and more importantly, what the long-term risks and complications are, given the child's present prognosis.

From my own experience as a student midwife, I know how easy it is for those who work in the intensive care environment to become so familiar with its day-to-day running, that they forget what a formidable place it looks to the layperson. Parents can be very easily intimidated by the technology, and may feel afraid to ask questions or raise concerns about treatment, because they feel staff are too busy to be interrupted. This is particularly true of young single parents, or those with a limited capacity for understanding medical jargon. They, too, have the right to expect simple, direct and understandable communication from the medical team, so that they feel that they are being listened to when decisions about their child are being made. Doctors or nurses who are used to dealing with emergency episodes can sometimes brush aside what appears to be a major crisis to the caring parent, as only a minor problem. Parents may, at this time, be frightened and bewildered about the infant's condition; staff need to talk them through the baby's diagnosis and prognosis and perhaps offer guidance in the face of what must seem a terrifying set of options. Nevertheless, from those who have spoken to me, it is obvious that parents feel better able to cope with whatever might happen in the future, if they know what to expect.

If the baby dies

> Normally, letting go is a drawn out process of trusting the child to find her own path through life, giving her room to grow into a responsible, independent person. Most parents have many years to give their child roots and wings. But when the letting go involves death, particularly so soon after birth, it can be incredibly difficult. It is just too soon.
>
> (Davis 2001, p. 2)

Generations ago, it was not unusual for almost every family to have experienced the death of at least one child, either at birth or in early infancy; and even if they had not experienced it themselves, they knew of a friend or neighbour who had suffered such a loss. Today, the death of a baby is less common. With high standards of antenatal care and the latest neonatal technology at our disposal, we have come to expect a trouble-free pregnancy resulting in the birth of a healthy baby. Even if things begin to go wrong, we may assume that modern medication and surgical skill will produce a good outcome.

The possibility of losing a baby at birth or shortly afterwards is something that is rarely mentioned at antenatal classes, or in any of the hundreds of books written about pregnancy and childbirth. It is natural in the months approaching birth that the medical team wish to engender a positive approach and not raise unnecessary worries, particularly with a first-time mother. However, it has been suggested that it may be a mistake to ignore the fact that a few parents will have to face the possibility of losing their baby. The death of their child is one of the worst nightmares any parent could anticipate, but it is a reality that some parents have to live with. Their baby may live for a few hours, a few days or a few weeks but in the end the infant may die unexpectedly, or perhaps even worse, a decision to withdraw treatment has to be made.

Many parents have described the hopes and happy anticipation that a very much longed for pregnancy brings. The excitement of making preparations: choosing names, planning the nursery, buying clothes and equipment, looking forward to finishing full-time work or maternity leave, meeting other parents-to-be at relaxation classes and antenatal clinics. After this, no parents are prepared for the devastation that comes when their new baby dies. One mother describes her feelings, which continued for many months after the death of her premature baby:

> Every night since then I've cried with sadness and guilt and sometimes anger. I keep going over and over the months I was pregnant, trying to think what I did wrong. I saw a psychiatrist for a few months but all he told me was to pull myself together, I wasn't the first woman to lose a baby and I wouldn't be the last. Besides I was only 20, I could have plenty more. But I don't want more, I want my son.
>
> (Kohner and Henley 2001, p. 19)

Deborah Davies is a psychologist who specialises in perinatal bereavement. In her work with parents of very premature babies, she has discovered that one of the main concerns for those forced to make the ultimate decision about whether or not to withdraw life support from their infant, is the amount of suffering their baby may have to endure while undergoing aggressive treatment in neonatal special care. Some of the parents that she has counselled decided to reject further medical intervention in favour of nursing care, allowing the child to die peacefully. They believed that the suffering far outweighed any possible benefits, either now or in the future. Davies (2001) emphasises that they chose this path, not because of any effect the child's disabilities might have on them or their family, but solely on the grounds of the misery the child was currently suffering and would continue to suffer throughout its life.

For these parents, Davies stresses the importance of pointing out that taking a decision of this kind is a great act of devotion. With their decision will have come feelings of guilt at the possibility that they have let the child down, or failed to protect them; they have abandoned a vulnerable child. It is important that they understand what a courageous and loving act it was; that the decision was made because they wanted what was best for their baby.

> The loss of a child is as bad as it gets in human experience. It is totally devastating in any circumstances.
>
> (Jean Simons, Daily Express, 8th January 2002, p. 3)

Grief for the death of a child evokes deep feelings of guilt, anger, fear and regret. Parents need to be reassured that these are natural reactions and they are not acting in an abnormal way. Some have said that friends, relatives and neighbours sometimes avoid talking about the tragedy because they find it hard to know what to say. The child's death also induces deep feelings within them, and they are unable to cope with the level of grief and desolation they know the parents must be feeling. They may feel deeply sympathetic, but at the same time almost frightened to approach the bereaved family. Many people who have lost children find this silence unbearable: they need to talk about their baby, to feel that they are being heard and that their loss is recognised. Some have expressed hurt and anger that close friends and family cannot understand why they continue to grieve many months later, assuming that if they 'try again' for another child, it will erase the memory of the dead baby. Somehow, because the baby was so young, they will get over the loss more quickly, or even forget the event altogether.

As most parents who have lost a baby at birth or shortly afterwards can confirm, they never 'get over' their loss. Like any other bereaved person, they may eventually come to terms and accept it; but as with the death of any other loved family member, they never forget or stop loving them. There is no time limit; as with everything else, mourning is an individual thing. People react in different ways and it is important that they are able to express their grief in whichever way helps them.

Some tell and retell the story; others visit and tend the grave frequently, sometimes on a daily basis: this gives them a focus and purpose and helps them feel closer to the dead baby. It is important that whichever coping mechanism is adopted, family and friends are supportive and uncritical. Choosing words for a memorial or scattering ashes can help in the process of 'letting go'.

However, even when they have been supported well, after a while some parents come to feel that they may need to have contact with others who have suffered similar bereavements and understand what they are going through. They may think that they cannot continue to burden their immediate family and friends with their grief any longer, so seek help from a more detached source, because they find it easier to talk to someone with whom they are not emotionally involved and who may help them see things from a different perspective. Bereavement counselling will give them the opportunity to express feelings that they may not be able to communicate to close family or friends, thus helping them come to terms with their grief.

In some cases, bereaved parents do not seek the help they need immediately, and never fully express their grief at the time of their loss. It may only become apparent months, even years after the baby's death that there are unresolved issues to be dealt with. Sometimes, perhaps at the time of a birthday or anniversary, strong emotions will surface and these may manifest themselves in a number of ways: overwhelming depression, marital conflict, or problems with other children in the family. Parents in this situation need to be reassured that these are common problems and help is available, however long it is since their loss.

Naturally, services vary from area to area; what is needed is a good information service that will help anyone find the appropriate kind of support they require.

Most maternity hospitals now run courses to train midwives as bereavement counsellors, whose role is to help parents whose baby has died.

Mothers who gave birth to premature babies years ago never had the chance to see them or hold them. They were whisked away immediately after delivery, to be disposed of without ceremony. At the time it was considered the kindest and best thing to do; but it is now known that many of these women and men, now in their sixties and seventies, bitterly regret not being given the opportunity of knowing how their offspring looked or of briefly touching them; they were denied the chance to say goodbye to the baby they had carried through pregnancy and whose birth had been eagerly anticipated.

Today, parents are given the choice about whether they wish to see their dead baby. Some choose not to, and their wishes are respected; but Kohner and Henley (2001) emphasise how important it is for hospitals to provide parents with as much help and information as possible at this time about the sorts of things they can do to build up positive memories of their child. Some parents are so shocked and grief stricken that they cannot think clearly about the choices they might make, and they often live to regret the fact that they never saw or held their child when they had the opportunity. One such parent described how she had been given the option immediately after birth, but had declined. It was only afterwards that she realised she'd made the wrong choice, and wished that someone had taken the time to explain to her about how saying goodbye would have helped with the grieving process.

Some parents appreciate the opportunity to share their grief. Some hospitals provide facilities; a side ward where they and their infant can be alone together or receive visitors. It is important for some that family and friends can come and see the baby and acknowledge them as parents. Research has shown that if they are encouraged to hold, cuddle and dress the child, as they would if he/she were alive, it acts as the initial step in helping them come to terms with the death. Many parents now testify to the significance of such practices. The fact that a mother or father knows they will never again have the opportunity to bathe and clothe their child gives them the opportunity of performing a family ritual just once.

It helps enormously in the grieving process if bereaved parents feel they are being treated with respect and given the right kind of support during their time in the hospital. Sensitive and compassionate care from staff before and after the child's death can help to alleviate the stress and pain that parents experience. Even though the child has died, parents need the reassurance of nurses and doctors that their baby is still important and that they still matter. It will not diminish their acute sense of loss, but the memory of feeling cared for by understanding professionals will always remain and serve as a positive remembrance in an otherwise traumatic episode.

Nowadays, a memory bank of photographs, footprints and handprints can be built up, and stored for future reference if parents are not ready to handle them and take them home immediately. Often, at a future date these mementoes may be claimed when the parents feel ready to deal with the painful memories and make closure complete.

Some parents choose to take their dead baby home, so that the whole family can express their grief in familiar surroundings. Although others might find this an abnormal thing to do, one mother felt that for her it was the most natural thing in the world. She expressed her feelings thus:

> You never imagine you'll be holding your dead baby; you recoil from the idea of it, but somehow when it happens to you, it's absolutely the right thing.
>
> (Joanna Moorhead 2002, p. 15)

Moorhead (2002) also reminds us that for those who have lost newborn babies, the complacency of pregnancy is lost forever. A further pregnancy only serves to magnify the fear that the same thing will happen again. Parental anxieties are increased; nothing is ever taken for granted again and even when things appear to be progressing normally, the health of the unborn baby is always a concern.

SUPPORT FOR STAFF IN NEONATAL CARE UNITS

Wyatt and Spencer (1992) believe that it is important to recognise the degree of emotional stress experienced by medical and nursing staff involved in the death of a baby in intensive care. They may have been engaged in the care and treatment of this baby for weeks, even months, and have formed a strong emotional tie with both child and family through the ups and downs of treatment. They too may feel that they have let the child down in some way. If death is the eventual outcome, it is easy to understand that nursing staff in particular may experience a sense of grief, frustration and sometimes guilt. Robertson (1998) believes that it can sometimes even affect the nurse's own attitudes to mothering or death.

Doctors have the difficult task of informing parents and dealing with whatever reactions may arise from their misery. This will require sensitive careful handling and may not come easily to some professionals, who find it a lonely and demanding duty. Summers (2002) points out that there are no private facilities in specialist units for very ill babies. Therefore the doctors who choose to work in neonatal intensive care have to be dedicated to working within the NHS and not looking for lucrative work in the private sector, which makes it a fairly unpopular choice of specialisation in medical terms.

Nevertheless, however distressing the situation may appear for medical staff, the very fact that they have chosen this work means that they accept certain responsibilities as part of their professional duty. At the same time, the pressures involved in working in such an atmosphere should not be dismissed as trivial. It is a highly demanding and specialised field and, according to Summers (2002), has a high rate of emotional and physical burnout. These nurses are no better paid than any others; they face short staffing and frequently are called upon to cover for each other.

For these reasons, many hospitals now recommend that a pastoral care team is available for any member of staff, giving them the time and opportunity to talk in private, and express any emotions that might emerge from a distressing situation. Alongside such facilities, it is essential that adequate training be provided so that every member of staff feels confident in their ability to offer appropriate support to family members and colleagues.

Mason and McCall Smith (1999) also emphasise the importance of considering the dilemmas of conscience that some staff involved in the process of withholding and withdrawing intensive treatment from neonates may have. They advocate that any proposed legislation should include clauses to safeguard the positions and sensitivities of nurses or health workers. They are the ones who bear the brunt of selective treatment decisions; therefore, their feelings should be considered and respected. A team approach is recommended, so that all opinions are heard, and this is increasingly becoming the accepted way forward in many neonatal intensive treatment units.

PART 2

The legal and ethical framework

Part 2 considers some key legal cases, codes of ethics and philosophical theories that underpin the process of decision-making in neonatal intensive care.

PART CONTENTS

6

The legal framework

> Laws are not the basis of medical ethics.
>
> (Gillon 1985, p. 13)

RELATIONSHIP BETWEEN ETHICS AND THE LAW

Although doctors are bound by the law and are obliged to practice within the law, laws can change rapidly. As Gillon (1985) points out, a practice deemed unprofessional or illegal can rapidly become both legal and acceptable. What is acceptable within the law of one culture may be completely illegal in another society.

When discussing the subject of ethics in general terms, we may be thinking of a code of conduct or a system of belief that can help individuals discriminate between 'right' and 'wrong'. This may or may not coincide with what is acceptable within the bounds of the law. Actions that some people would consider morally wrong are not necessarily against the law.

Sometimes individuals or groups deliberately and publicly disobey the law on a matter of principle, because they feel morally bound to challenge it. One such confrontation between the law and ethics occurred when the 1967 Abortion Act was introduced. There were massive demonstrations by Pro Life groups opposed on ethical grounds to any such legislation. Although the Act was passed, and abortion is no longer illegal, many people believe that it is unethical.

In the first part of this section I want to look at aspects of the law that relate to the problems surrounding the saving of very premature babies, along with some relevant cases; in the second part I will examine some of the theories and principles which help doctors and ethicists in the decision-making process.

The law

> Despite the plethora of new ethical problems created daily by modern medicine and the changed moral climate, the law remains relatively unchanged. No statute expressly addresses the fate of the newborn infant with multiple handicap who in an earlier age would have died whatever had been done for her.
>
> (Brazier 1992, p. 39)

According to Kennedy and Grubb (1995) English law is committed to the sanctity of life principle. They emphasise that courts will always strongly presume in favour of taking every possible step to preserve life, and would never sanction steps to terminate it, even for those children with overwhelming disabilities. However, they do concede that, in certain circumstances, other competing principles may have to be considered. Problems arise when trying to recognise those circumstances, and to identify which other principles may be relevant.

It is generally assumed that a child under the age of 12 years is not sufficiently mature to make decisions about consenting or withholding consent for medical treatment. As we have seen, one of the dilemmas in the treatment of children, particularly those infants born prematurely and/or with multiple disabilities, has been created by the availability of sophisticated, life-saving technology. Differences can emerge about who is in the best position to make the crucial decisions about the use of this technology on behalf of the infant: the medical team have knowledge and expertise, but the parents are ultimately responsible for caring for the child, who may be severely disabled. What happens if these two cannot agree on the best course of treatment? How can the best interests of the child be protected in law?

Whatever their ethical stand on matters relating to the treatment of babies born with multiple physical and mental disabilities, both doctors and parents have certain legal obligations which limit their actions and choices in relation to the care of the child.

Criminal law and the duty of care

Montgomery (1997) explains that in law, doctors have a duty of care to their patients, and parents have a duty of care to their children.

> Consequently, the parties involved in deciding what care a newborn baby should receive may be bound to take active steps to care for the child and can be held responsible for failing to act, as well as for taking positive steps to kill. Liability turns on the extent of the duty to take active steps.
>
> (Montgomery 1997, p. 412)

It appears that the parents' 'reasonable actions' and the professionals' 'proper practice' are the acceptable boundaries governing what the law regards as acceptable care. Of course, there may be wide interpretations of what could be regarded as a 'reasonable action' on the part of the parent, and even more scope when deciding what is 'proper practice' on the medical side.

In a simple case of caring parents trying to do their best for their sick child, Brazier (1992) tells us that as far as consent is concerned, their authority is acceptable in law.

However, problems with consent may arise if a parent is not on hand at the time of an emergency; for example if a child is involved in an accident and needs urgent treatment or life-saving surgery. In these circumstances a doctor will be protected in law if he gives whatever treatment he deems appropriate and necessary, in the knowledge that it is what any reasonable and concerned parent would wish him to do. Indeed, if he did not act in this way, he may find himself guilty of criminal neglect.

What if a parent is available, but appears indifferent to the child's welfare; or if they fail to turn up after being contacted about the child's whereabouts and condition? Again, in either of these two situations, the doctor would be within his rights to treat the child in whatever way he feels is in its best interests.

The biggest dilemma is caused when parents refuse consent for the course of action proposed by doctors; as, for example, in the case of a Jehovah's Witness who refuses to give consent for a life-saving blood transfusion for a critically ill child. Brazier (1992) maintains that in an emergency situation, when immediate treatment is required, the doctor could overrule the wishes of the parents and still be protected in law, even without having to resort to applying for the child to be made a ward of court. The medical defence for this position would be to state that parents have a duty to provide adequate medical care for the child, and that anyone who fails in this duty can be charged with wilful neglect. These points are all made clear in legislation:

- **The Children and Young Persons' Act 1933**. Parents are required to do whatever is 'reasonable' to safeguard and promote their children's welfare, risking prosecution for child neglect if they do not provide adequate medical care for them. What is regarded as a 'reasonable action' on the part of the parents may be open to interpretation. In law, however, it does seem that this is interpreted as 'acting as any reasonable parent would do in the circumstances'. Reasonable action could involve consenting or withholding consent; but as Montgomery (1997) further points out, where parents decide against treatment, it would be difficult to prove their action 'unreasonable' if they believed they were acting in their child's best interests.
- **The Children Act 1989**. The paramount consideration enshrined within this legislation is the welfare of children within all court decisions. Both doctors and parents are bound to consider the best interests of the child at all times. If doctor and parents disagree about a course of action and parental consent is withheld, the doctor can overrule the parents' decision if he deems that intervention is both urgent and necessary. Sometimes, a care and protection order can be put into place if the parents are strongly opposed to the doctor's proposed treatment. On the

other hand, the Act could uphold the parental wishes and rights, but only if the medical team are in agreement that the treatment is not necessary. So, as Brazier (1992) points out, the criminal law will only take into account what is objectively considered medically necessary, and will not necessarily be swayed by the personal views and values of parents. In the vast majority of cases, the child's best interests are represented by loving and caring parents, and their views may not lightly be disregarded when they conflict with those of the doctor. However, in the final analysis, if the child's best interests appear to be represented by the doctor, then parental wishes will be overridden. Doctors are also liable to prosecution if they bring about the death of a child by any active intervention. On the other hand, if they withhold life-saving treatment, the position in law is less clear. The trial of Dr Leonard Arthur in 1981, described later in this section, illustrates the competing principles which must be considered.

- **The European Convention on Human Rights**. It is now necessary to consider implications arising from this statute which came into force in Great Britain in 2000 and which reiterates British criminal law. Article 2 states:

> Everyone's right to life shall be protected by law. No one shall be deprived of his life intentionally.

KILLING OR ALLOWING TO DIE: IS THERE A DIFFERENCE IN LAW?

In English law a crime is viewed from two perspectives:

- **The forbidden situation**: Which means, what the accused actually did.
- **The state of mind of the accused at the time of the offence**: This involves the *intention* of the accused and not their *motive* for committing the crime. If the killing of a patient is intentional, for whatever reason, then the crime is murder, and the sentence is mandatory life imprisonment. Therefore, even though a doctor may have acted with the best of motives, a deliberate act of 'mercy killing' to end the life of a patient suffering from an agonising terminal illness would still leave him open to a murder charge. It makes no difference whether the patient has begged for help to die more quickly, euthanasia is still illegal under English law.

The doctrine of acts and omissions

Having described these two perspectives, it must be emphasised that legally a distinction is drawn between when a person acts and when a person fails to act. As we have seen, in English law, if a death is caused by an intentional act, then there is no defence. Any motive for the killing is irrelevant. If a doctor intentionally causes the death of a patient, regardless of their motive, they are guilty of murder. On the other hand, if the death is caused by a doctor *omitting* to act, he or she may not necessarily be held liable (Ferguson 1997).

So where does this leave the treatment of the critically ill neonate in relation to the law? It is obvious that these patients lack the capacity to speak for themselves, but more than that, some would argue that they are also patients for whom no 'substituted judgement' can be given, because their past and present wishes cannot possibly be known. They have no autonomy and in law are considered incompetent (Campbell and McHaffie 1995).

In these circumstances, how is the doctor to interpret his 'duty of care' and proper practice? Will the withdrawal of life support, in the belief that it is in the best interest of his patient, be seen as a deliberate and intended action? If so, he may leave himself open to an accusation of intending to bring about a death, and find himself on a murder charge.

> A baby is born with severe disabilities and the decision is made that in the child's best interests it would be advisable not to ventilate. Eventually the infant develops a chest infection, but no antibiotics are prescribed, so he dies. It can be argued legally that by doing nothing actively to bring about the death of the child, but doing nothing to prevent it either, 'nature was allowed to take its course'.
>
> (Kuhse and Singer 1985, p. 80)

In this case, although the doctor knows that if he does not intervene with life-saving treatment, the child will almost certainly die, he would defend his decision on the grounds that he was acting in the child's best interests. The baby was not capable of independent existence; therefore, it died of natural causes. Because of the massive damage sustained at birth its prognosis was extremely poor; aggressive treatment could not improve the situation but only add to the distress already suffered. In other words, the clinical assessment was not to intervene, and to allow the infant to die in peace.

Certainly, the interpretation of 'the child's best interest' in the English courts appears to revolve around the likely degree of suffering that the child will be expected to bear. In other words, future quality of life has the capacity to influence a court's ruling.

The doctrine of double effect

> There is a difference between what one aims at (one's direct intention) and what is foreseen but is not intended (one's oblique intention).
>
> (Singleton and McLaren 1995, p. 60)

This principle can be seen operating when a doctor knowingly administers a massive dose of a pain-killing drug to someone who is terminally ill, in the knowledge that this may speed up the death of the patient. Ferguson (1997) describes the case of Dr John Bodkin Adams, who was accused of murder after administering a large dose of heroin and morphine to an eighty-one year old stroke victim. The prosecution maintained that if he knew the drugs would result in her death, then it could be said that he intended to kill her. However, the judge directed the jury that the doctor was acting in a proper and necessary way to relieve pain and suffering, even though the measures he took incidentally shortened her life. The doctor was said to be acting in the best interest of his patient.

What if an infant resuscitated at birth and kept alive by invasive and artificial means is later discovered to be suffering from profound neurological damage? A decision by doctors to withdraw life support could be supported by arguing that the action was taken in order to alleviate further suffering and distress to the infant. His death may have been *foreseen* as a consequence of the action, but the primary *intention* was to save him from further invasive and traumatic treatment, which would have been futile in the long term.

This is a fine distinction, the ethics of which are discussed in the section in this book on withdrawing and withholding treatment.

Sanctity of life versus quality of life

According to Kennedy and Grubb (1995) English law is committed to the sanctity of life principle. They emphasise that courts will always strongly presume in favour of taking every possible step to preserve life, and would never sanction steps to terminate it, even for those children with overwhelming disabilities.

However, they do concede that sometimes other competing principles may have to be considered.

> In so far as the tradition has been for the courts in the United Kingdom to allow themselves to be led by the medical profession, it is not necessarily surprising that both appear to pay lip service to the sanctity of life, while leaving a vast discretion to the doctor in charge, in consultation with the parents.
>
> (Wells 1989, p. 209)

The *quality of life* principle seems most pertinent in most court decisions.

SOME RELEVANT CASES

Re B 1981 (Montgomery, 1997)

The parents of a Down's Syndrome baby refused consent to surgery for intestinal obstruction, feeling that it would be better for the child to be allowed to die. As Montgomery points out, if the child had not been suffering from Down's Syndrome, there would have been no hesitation in performing the surgery. Doctors disagreed with the parental decision and the child was made a ward of court. The counsel for the parents presented them as a responsible and caring couple whose wishes should be respected; nevertheless, their plea was rejected as not being in the child's best interests. The Court of Appeal authorised the operation because the judge deemed that there was no evidence that her life was so 'demonstrably awful' that she should be left to die. The implication here seems to be that withholding treatment from any child is not justifiable in law unless the courts can be certain that the child's future will be so full of pain and suffering as to be deemed 'not worth living'.

Re C 1989 (Campbell and McHaffie, 1995)

The child was born at 27 weeks' gestation and suffered multiple disabilities because of complications arising from low birth weight and prematurity. At sixteen weeks she had severe cerebral palsy, and was blind and hydrocephalic. The prognosis was that she would eventually die. The court was asked to decide, firstly, whether she should be treated with antibiotics if she developed an infection and, secondly, whether she should be fed by nasogastric tube or intravenously if she could no longer be fed by syringe. The judge considered that, as the child's death was anticipated anyway, the judgement turned on relieving the suffering of the child for as long as was necessary. He advised that those caring for her should not be *obliged* to resort to artificial feeding or prescribing antibiotics and permitted the hospital authority liberty to treat the baby in a manner which would allow her life to end peacefully and with dignity (Brazier, 1992).

Re J 1990 (Brazier 1992)

A baby boy, born thirteen weeks premature with very low birth weight, suffered several major setbacks, each one treated by aggressive intervention. The result was that the child suffered massive brain damage. The future prognosis indicated that multiple disabilities were foreseen, but unlike the case of Re C, none of these disabilities were life threatening in the short term. The court was asked to consider what should be done if at some point he needed antibiotics, and whether, if he suffered further collapse, he should be resuscitated. In his judgement, at the Court of Appeal, Lord Donaldson held that the withholding of treatment for a severely handicapped baby was justified when the future quality of life would be intolerable. In his statement he said:

> In the end there will be cases in which the answer must be that it is not in the interests of the child to subject it to treatment which will cause increased suffering and produce no commensurate benefit, giving the fullest possible weight to the child's and mankind's desire to survive.
>
> (Brazier 1992, p. 323)

Re C (a baby) 1996 (Mason and McCall Smith, 2000)

This case involved a premature baby girl who suffered meningitis resulting in blindness, deafness and frequent convulsions. She was kept alive on life support and it was thought that she could continue living in this way for up to two years. Although she was not unconscious, her level of awareness was extremely low and not expected to improve. In the meantime, it was anticipated that her suffering would get worse and her existence was described as a 'living death'. Doctors confirmed that she was not capable of independent existence and that withdrawing ventilation would mean that death would occur within hours. It was the opinion of both doctors and parents that it would be in the baby's best interests to discontinue life support and permission was granted to follow this course of action.

Re J (a minor) (medical treatment) 1993 (Mason and McCall Smith, 2000)

A child sustained massive brain damage following an accident. Although medical opinion considered intensive care treatment to be futile, the mother insisted that doctors try to save her son. A Court of Appeal upheld the doctors' clinical decision and refused to direct them to provide treatment against their better judgement. This case once again shows that quality of life issues tend to be favoured over the idea that life must be preserved at all costs. It also confirms the view that courts almost always find in favour of medical opinion and a doctor's clinical autonomy.

Re v Arthur 12 BMLRI 1981 (Montgomery, 1997)

A baby with Down's Syndrome was rejected by his mother immediately following birth. Subsequently, both parents expressed a wish for the child to be allowed to die. Dr Leonard Arthur, a well-known paediatrician, concurred and prescribed a drug to suppress the child's appetite. He ordered that the child should be hydrated, but not fed, with nursing care only. The child died three days later. A pro-life group prosecuted the doctor and initially the charge was murder. However, after a post-mortem, it was found that the child had more complications than was at first thought and would have died anyway, so the charge was reduced to attempted murder. The prosecution's case made it clear that, at the time he prescribed the drugs, Dr Arthur was not aware of any other medical problems, and other witnesses supported the view that there was no reason for him to prescribe them in such huge doses. The key question was whether Dr Arthur intended to kill the baby, or whether he had simply not *intervened* to prolong its life. Several witnesses for the defence stated that the doctor's actions constituted normal medical practice, and the court accepted their statements. Despite reminding the jury of the difference between motive and intent, and also insisting that when the law and ethics are in conflict, then the law must always prevail, the judge then proceeded to make his final, contradictory, summary. "I imagine that you [the jury], will think long and hard before deciding that doctors of the eminence we have heard representing to you what medical ethics are and apparently have been for over a period of time, you will think long and hard before concluding that they in that great profession have evolved standards which amount to committing a crime" (Brazier 1992, p. 317). Dr Leonard Arthur was acquitted.

Scotland: The case of baby Cassidy

In 1996 a baby girl of 23 weeks' gestation and weighing 1lb 4oz was born to Kirsty Cassidy in a Scottish hospital. Doctors immediately assessed that the baby was 'not viable' and decided not to perform aggressive treatment. Kirsty disagreed and wished for her daughter to be given a chance of life, however slim. Her wishes were ignored and the baby died in her arms. Mrs Cassidy demanded an inquiry, saying that her wishes had been ignored and that the doctors had acted unlawfully in leaving her baby to die. In June 1997 the Sheriff's Court in Kilmarnock rejected her plea, and announced that the hospital had acted in the infant's best interests, by saving her from painful and invasive intervention.

USA: The case of baby Messenger

In February 1994 a baby boy of only 25 weeks' gestation, weighing 1lb 12oz, was born to Traci and Gregory Messenger in Lansing, Michigan. The parents at once decided that the chances of severe disability were too high to risk aggressive treatment and requested that their baby be allowed to die peacefully. The medical team disagreed, and the child was taken immediately to neonatal intensive care for resuscitation. When the child was one hour old, Gregory Messenger, himself a doctor, disconnected his son from the ventilator and gave him to his mother to cuddle. The tiny baby died in her arms. Doctors at the hospital gave the cause of death as 'homicide'. Dr Messenger was sent for trial and the courts were asked to consider whether he had left his son to die unlawfully. In February 1995, Dr Messenger was acquitted of manslaughter.

RE A (CHILDREN): THE CASE OF THE CONJOINED TWINS, JODIE AND MARY

The final case we will consider here will be covered in more detail. It caught the public interest and is unusual in that it deals with the lives of not one child, but two; nevertheless the legal and ethical implications in the judgement are just as relevant, no matter how many babies are involved. The case was extremely complicated and caused even the judges involved some sleepless nights. The following account is based on an article (Mifflin, 2001) I wrote for a journal, *The Practising Midwife*, which helps illustrate some of the very complex ethical issues thrown up by this legal battle.

Background to the case

The parents were flown to the UK on May 16th 2000 from the tiny island of Gozo, after it was discovered that the mother was pregnant with conjoined twins.

They were brought to St Mary's Hospital in Manchester by means of a shared quota arrangement between the National Health Service and the Maltese health authorities, because of the lack of appropriate facilities at home. However, it was soon discovered that the because of the nature and extent of the foetal abnormalities, surgery was out of the question during pregnancy.

The clinical condition and prognosis after birth

The baby girls were born by caesarean section on August 8th 2000 and both required immediate resuscitation. To safeguard their anonymity they were given false names of Jodie and Mary.

The twins were joined at the lower abdomen, having a fused spine with interchange of spinal fluid. Their legs were splayed out sideways, Jodie's to the left and Mary's to the right. The bladder, rectum, anal and genital areas were shared, as were their digestive and circulatory systems, including surrounding tissue and muscle. Most significantly, they shared two major blood vessels, the aorta and vena cava.

Mary's heart and lungs soon became non-functional, so that she relied completely on Jodie's heart and lungs for oxygen and nutrients. This placed Jodie's organs under immense pressure, ensuring that if nothing were done, both babies would die within six months.

Jodie was described as 'bright and alert' and although further major reconstructive surgery was foreseen, it was felt that she had a good chance of survival if separated from Mary.

Mary was badly brain damaged, but sucking reflex and arm movements were present.

The dilemma

The medical team knew that if they did nothing both children would die within six months but if surgery was commenced, clamping of the aorta would mean immediate death for Mary. Could they justify sacrificing one child in order to save the other? On balance, they recommended that surgery be undertaken.

The twins' parents are devout Roman Catholics and hold very strong moral and religious views. Because they loved both children equally they felt it would be absolutely wrong to sacrifice the life of one of their babies, even though it meant saving the other. Their view was that it was the future of the babies was in God's hands, and they expressed the wish to let 'nature take its course'.

As a result of this impasse, the hospital decided to ask the courts to uphold the recommendations of the doctors and overrule the wishes of the parents.

The legal battle

The case was heard on August 25th 2000 in the Family Division of the High Court where permission was given to the hospital for the separation of the twins.

The parents, supported by the Roman Catholic church and pro-life groups, launched an appeal to stop the surgery, which began on 4th September and was to become unique in legal history.

The case raised acute legal and ethical issues. Would Mary's death be an intentional killing, and if so, were the doctors guilty of murder? Is one life more valuable than another? Does everyone have a moral right to life?

The courts acknowledged the terrible dilemma the parents had to face and said that they had listened to their plea and accepted their moral argument. However, those wishes were overruled on the grounds that ethically, separation of the twins would be 'the lesser of two evils'.

There were those who questioned this decision, making the point that parents are not usually deprived of the authority to make health care decisions on behalf of their children unless they are proved to be either incompetent or negligent. This did not apply in this case, and parental wishes were established as morally acceptable; so, it was argued, the courts should have allowed the parents to determine the outcome.

Lord Justice Ward made the point that the best interests of the child are always paramount in family law, but that courts could not approve a course of action which may be illegal. Arising from this, he concluded there arose four crucial issues:

1. Is it in Jodie's best interests that she be separated from Mary?
2. Is it in Mary's best interests that she be separated from Jodie?
3. If those interests are in conflict, can the court balance the interests of one against the other and so allow one to prevail against the other and, if that is permissible, how is that balancing exercise to be undertaken?
4. If the prevailing interest is in favour of the operation being performed, can it be lawfully performed?

Interestingly, under the Children Act, there are no provisions for dealing with such a situation. The rights of the child are always paramount when set against other criteria, but when the rights of two children conflict, there is nothing in law that gives guidance as to whose rights should take precedence.

Jodie's best interests

Taking the first of the points raised above, the comments of Lord Justice Ward summed up the conclusions reached by all three Appeal Court judges, saying that it would be "overwhelmingly in her [Jodie's] interest that she be given the chance to live a normal life, with a normal expectation of life. It is certainly not in her best interest to be left to die." Evidence suggested that because of Mary's conjoined existence, she posed a serious threat to the life of Jodie and therefore Jodie was entitled to protest that Mary was killing her, by inadvertently using her organs and eventually causing her death. Mary was presented as an 'unintentional aggressor' and it is legitimate in law to kill another person, even a child, if one is acting in self-defence. Obviously, in this case Jodie could not act for herself, therefore it would be acceptable that her doctors should come to her aid and remove the threat (i.e. Mary), which was draining away her life.

Mary's best interests

Before the second question could be answered a preliminary legal issue needed to be settled: was Mary a live person in her own right, or was she (as had been implied by some), more like a tumour or a parasite, which of course would have no legal status? Medical evidence was overwhelming in confirming that Mary was indeed a person in her own right, and therefore entitled to all the rights and protection that the law could offer.

Lord Justice Ward, speaking for all three judges, confirmed that surgery would not be in Mary's best interests, for it would inevitably result in her death. Counsel defending Mary's case argued, firstly, that the sanctity of life doctrine dictated that Mary's life was of equal value in law to that of her sister; secondly, that if human life is inviolable, then it would be wrong to cause the death of an innocent person by act or omission; and thirdly, that it is wrong to invade anyone's bodily integrity, knowing that the consequences would be of no benefit to that person. In Mary's case, it could only result in death.

Weighing the balance

Despite the fact that all the above points were upheld, the judges decided that it was impossible to make a judgement about the worthwhileness of Mary's life against that of Jodie; instead they needed to look at the worthwhileness of the treatment — in other words, what kind of life each twin could expect to enjoy if separation took place. This perspective brought into play the quality of life versus sanctity of life issues which so often influence a court's decisions and, of course, the balance weighed heavily against Mary. In the words of Lord Justice Ward:

> The sad fact is that Mary lives on borrowed time, all of it borrowed from her sister. She is incapable of independent existence, she is designated for death.

Can the operation be performed legally?

Those against the operation felt that rather than trying to protect Mary's rights, the courts had seemed to concentrate more on finding ways to justify her killing. The ProLife Alliance stated: "How to turn an unlawful killing into a lawful killing: that was the question." They went on to warn of the 'slippery slope' argument: "If we can kill Mary, why not any other newborn baby with a poor prognosis?" The court acknowledged that the case was harrowing and unique, and that the decision reached was not one of right versus wrong, but that it was a choice between the 'lesser of two evils'. They concluded that doctors carrying out the operation would commit no unlawful act because, firstly, the exceptional circumstances of the case justified the plea that they were acting on Jodie's behalf to remove the threat of fatal harm, and secondly, although the operation would involve a positive act of invasive surgery, and the death of Mary would be foreseen as a consequence, the primary intention of the surgeons would be to save the life of Jodie.

The verdict

The court's verdict on 22nd September 2000 was to dismiss the appeal and allow the operation to take place. The parents were urged to take their case to the House of Lords, but declined, finally accepting the judges' decision. Surgery was undertaken in early November, when the twins were three months old. The operation lasted twenty hours. Mary, as expected, did not survive. Jodie survived and was eventually allowed out of hospital to go back to Gozo with her parents. Doctors said that she had a good chance of living a normal life. However, it is thought that she will need to undergo several further operations to achieve this goal.

WHAT IMPLICATIONS CAN BE DRAWN FROM THESE CASES?

In Brazier's view, the interpretation of the child's 'best interests' is the crucial issue in cases like these. In English courts, interpretation of 'best interests' appears to revolve around the likely degree of suffering the child will be expected to bear. In other words, future quality of life has the capacity to influence a court's ruling.

Both parents and medical staff must be seen in law to be working for the child's best interests. The parents cannot be seen to have any selfish motives when deciding whether to withdraw or withhold treatment for their baby. Their wishes are not conclusive and can be overruled by a doctor, if he believes he may be acting unlawfully by withholding treatment. But doctors must not be seen to be over-zealous, treating babies for the sake of furthering their knowledge and experience, even though the expertise gained would benefit children in the future. The object of treatment must be to allow the child to die with minimum suffering.

At the beginning of this section, I quoted experts who maintain that English law is committed to upholding the sanctity of life principle at all times. The cases detailed above demonstrate that quality of life considerations play a major part in court decisions. It is also the case that the law in England has generally upheld medical decisions that have been challenged in court.

Some believe that society should be offering clearer guidelines in these muddied waters; others feel that too much rigidity in the law could create even more problems. Doctors in the USA believe that they have to treat all terminally ill babies with aggressive and futile treatment, or risk prosecution for neglect.

In the UK, the medical profession has introduced guidelines designed to help doctors solve the complexities of decision making when confronted by such dilemmas, and to help regulate practice when treating vulnerable groups.

Guidelines issued by the Ethics Advisory Committee of the Royal College of Paediatrics and Child Health (RCPCH 1997)

- **Section 2.3.1.2** states that under The Children Act 1989, the child's welfare is paramount. It also recognises the responsibility of parents to make decisions on behalf of their children, so accepting that joint medical and parental decisions are the most desirable and parental authority is to be sought at all times. However it also reiterates that parental authority can be overruled if a doctor is clearly acting in the child's best interests.
- **Section 2.7.1** describes quality of life criteria which may render a child's life 'not worth living'; while at the same time recognising

that what could be considered intolerable for a previously able bodied person would not necessarily be considered so by someone who has been born disabled.

• **Section 3.1.3** contains guidance for the withdrawal or withholding of treatment while still operating within the bounds of the law. In a 'no hope/no chance' situation, where treatment is only delaying death and not actually improving the quality or potential of the child's life, the doctor is under no legal obligation to provide any treatment if it is not in the best interest of his patient. Indeed, deliberate futile treatment it may constitute an assault. In a 'no purpose' situation, the prognosis is for an 'impossibly poor life', either in the future, in which case treatment might not be initiated, or in the present, with the likelihood of it continuing with no foreseeable improvement. In either case, treatment might reasonably be withdrawn. The example given is of a neonate with profound neurological damage, following severe asphyxia, where microcephaly, profound developmental delay, blindness and quadriplegia are believed to be inevitable.

Mason and McCall Smith (1999) argue that British doctors need more official guidance and protection under the law when they take on the responsibility of selective treatment in neonatal units. They claim that there is now sufficient case law to justify non-treatment decisions, and that although guidelines are in place, and doctors who knowingly ignore them will sometimes face the consequences, these are not legally binding, so cannot fully protect either doctor or patient.

Proposals for future legislation

Proposals for legislation on neonaticide have been introduced by those who are concerned to gain some clarification in law for the protection of doctors, and in response to concerns that babies who are grossly disabled should not be kept alive indefinitely, when their suffering and quality of life is too poor to be endured. The Limitation of Treatment Bill was proposed by two lawyers, Diana and Malcolm Brahams, and suggested that no criminal offence would be committed when a doctor refused or withdrew treatment from a neonate under the age of 28 weeks providing that (a) the parents gave written consent and (b) two doctors (one a paediatrician), both of at least seven years standing, certified in writing that the infant was suffering profound physical or mental handicap that was either irreversible or of such magnitude that the child could not enjoy any worthwhile quality of life, even after receiving every available treatment. In assessing the likely quality of life a number of factors were proposed for consideration, including the degree of pain and suffering the child was likely to suffer, his/her potential to communicate, parental willingness to care for the child and the effect that caring for the child could have on their physical and mental health.

Mason and McCall Smith (1999) point out the difficulties of positive legislation in the field of neonatal non-treatment, but do emphasise the need for more clarification within the law in order to protect doctors from accusations of deliberately killing infants. They propose the following clause, were such legislation to be brought onto the statute book:

> In the event of positive treatment being necessary for a neonate's survival, it will not be an offence to withhold such treatment if two doctors, one of whom is a consultant paediatrician, acting in good faith and with the consent of both parents if available, decide against treatment in the light of a reasonably clear medical prognosis which indicates that the infant's further life would be intolerable by virtue of pain or suffering or because of severe cerebral incompetence.
>
> (Mason and McCall Smith 1999, p. 390)

7

The ethical framework

Any action taken by an individual, a group or even society in general is ethical only if it protects the rights of those same individuals, groups or society. Ethical issues involve decisions about how we should or should not behave. They consider the norms and values of society; what actions are considered good and bad, right or wrong and what individuals should and should not do.

PROFESSIONAL CODES OF ETHICS

Most professional bodies are generally defined by their own codes of ethics, which inform members what is expected of them; and as Prichard (1996) points out, if someone is not prepared to comply with those requirements, then they forfeit their right of membership. She is sceptical of codes that set out to comply only with the written law, for morality is not just about sticking to rules, but about the way we think and behave within a particular profession.

> Indeed it can be said that it is a great failing of many so-called codes of ethics or practice that they merely set out what an employer is legally obliged to do... For a code to succeed as a moral document it must somehow advise and support its readers to behave in a way in which the Professional body at least, will recognise as good behaviour.
> (Pritchard 1996, p. 199)

Sim (1997) points out that individuals within a profession draw up professional codes of ethics, these codes have important implications for people outside the profession too: namely clients, patients and families. One of the problems associated with this is that representatives of the profession as a whole do not usually contribute to the construction of codes of ethics. It is senior members who are no longer practising who are often responsible for this, and their values may not reflect those of more junior colleagues, who are still working at a practical level. Also, they may not represent the views of society as a whole.

Medicine, of course, has its own code of ethics that had its origins in ancient Greek civilisation and is still referred to today as The Hippocratic Oath.

The Hippocratic Oath and its amendments

> I swear by Apollo the physician, and Aesculapius and Health, and all-hel, and all the gods and goddesses, that, according to my ability and judgement, I will keep this Oath.
>
> (Singleton and McLaren, 1995, p. 164)

Hippocrates (460-370BC) was a Greek philosopher, born on the island of Cos and known as 'The Father of Medicine'. His school of thought gave rise to a set of principles, formulated over 2500 years ago, that over the centuries have been interpreted and used as a basis for what we now refer to as the Hippocratic Oath. Over the past fifty years, advances in techniques, skills and equipment have given rise to moral and ethical problems that were unthinkable when the Oath was first devised. So, although some aspects of the code are still applicable and unchanged, underpinning the foundation for medical professional conduct and the doctor/patient relationship, others (some of which have a bearing on the issues surrounding the foetus, the neonate and sanctity of life issues) have been revoked or amended over the years.

The World Medical Association met in Geneva in 1948 to modernise the Hippocratic Oath. It was again amended, in Stockholm, in 1994 (see below), where some of the wording in relation to respect for human life was subtly changed from "I will maintain the utmost respect for human life, from the time of conception", to "I will maintain utmost respect for human life from its beginning." This fine difference in language has created a major debate about when human life actually begins.

Basic principles of the Hippocratic Oath

The doctor owes loyalty to his teachers and his brethren. It is interesting to note that the Oath names the doctor's first priority as loyalty to his 'teachers and brethren' not to his patients; the resonance of which seems to have been carried over the centuries and can still be detected in the close professional bond that exists between members of the profession. Nevertheless, in the Declaration of Geneva this clause is split: respect and gratitude to teachers comes second on the list and acknowledgment of colleagues as brothers and sisters is moved down to seventh place.

Obligations to exercise skill for the benefit of the patient. AB Shaw writes (1999) that Hippocrates recognised the duty of the doctor to his patient alone, but his oath would have been different if he had faced eight patients needing his four-bedded intensive care unit!

Abortion, direct euthanasia and abetting suicide are prohibited. Euthanasia and assisted suicide are still unlawful in this country and most others; one exception is the Northern Territory of Australia which passed legislation in 1995 to legalise voluntary euthanasia. However, as Mason and McCall (1999) point out the Hippocratic Oath may bar euthanasia as forbidden practice, but it does not impose any obligation to provide treatment at all times. Rather, it recommends an alternative and more pragmatic approach: 'Make a habit of two things – to help, or at least to do no harm', which today is interpreted in *The International Code of Medical Ethics* as 'acting in the best interest of the patient' or for their benefit. This of course can be interpreted in any number of ways; in the case of the very ill premature neonate, it could mean decisions immediately after birth about whether to begin or withhold life support; or later if treatment is futile, whether to withdraw or continue ventilation.

In both cases the dying child would be given palliative care, because any further 'extraordinary' treatment would be doing more harm than good.

Abortion, which is strictly forbidden in the Hippocratic Code, has now been legalised in many countries including Britain. Mason and McCall believe that the 1967 Abortion Act and the

Human Fertilisation and Embryology Act 1990 (Section 37) acted as a watershed, changing doctors' attitudes in relation to all aspects of life and death. These two Acts have made it fairly straightforward for a woman to obtain a termination of pregnancy up to the 24th week of pregnancy; and even after that it is also now possible, on certain grounds. After the 24th week there must be:

> • A risk of grave permanent injury to the physical or mental health of the pregnant woman.
> • That the continuation of the pregnancy would involve risk to the life of the pregnant woman, greater than if the pregnancy were terminated.
> • There is a substantial risk that if the child were born it would suffer such physical or mental abnormalities as to be severely handicapped.
> (Mason and McCall Smith 1999, p. 115)

A doctor should live a moral and upright life: Improper sexual relations with patients are banned. This clause has remained virtually unchanged. In *The International Code of Medical Ethics* the first duty of the doctor is to 'always maintain the highest standards of professional conduct'.

Confidentiality for patients was essential. Another interesting aspect of the code was the confidentiality clause; doctors have the privilege of being trusted with knowledge about patients, so must promise to use the knowledge solely for the good of that patient.

As Brazier (1992) writes, doctors, like priests should be able to keep secrets. Patients must have confidence that their doctor will not divulge any information that they give to him during a consultation; and in today's directives the doctor's duty is to promise to keep any confidences entrusted to him even after the patient's death.

However, although under the Hippocratic Oath doctors were obligated to keep their patients' confidences, they were not obliged to be truthful with them. On the contrary, they were strongly *discouraged* to be open and frank in their dealings:

> Concealing most things from the patient, while you were attending to him... turning his attention away from what is being done to him; ... revealing nothing of the patient's future or present condition.
> (Jennifer Jackson 2001, p. 11)

We can still see the influence of this in some doctors' approach to patients, and indeed in the way many patients still feel towards their doctor; even with the creation of the Patients' Charter and emphasis on patient autonomy, sometimes there is still a sense of deference towards one's physician and a sense that they know best. Campbell, Gillett and Jones (2001) describe it thus:

> Nevertheless the doctor is often still invested with a God-like authority, and faith in the doctor's ability to diagnose correctly and to prescribe effective treatment can be seen as an important component in the healing process.
>
> (Campbell, Gillett and Jones 2001, p. 21)

Jackson (2001) does believe that the directive in the Hippocratic Oath was made out of concern for the patient. It was meant in the best tradition of paternalism; to act in the most helpful way for the patient.

The Hippocratic Oath amended: The Declaration of Geneva International Code of Medical Ethics (amended in Stockholm 1994) (Mason and McCall Smith, p. 552)

When a doctor is admitted into the medical profession he/she makes these promises:

- I solemnly pledge myself to consecrate my life to the service of humanity;
- I will give to my teachers the respect and gratitude which is their due;
- I will practice my profession with conscience and dignity;
- The health of my patient will be my first consideration;
- I will respect the secrets which are confided in me, even after the patient has died;
- I will maintain by all means in my power, the honour and the noble traditions of the medical profession;
- My colleagues will be my sisters and brothers;
- I will not permit considerations of age, disease or disability, creed ethnic origin, gender, nationality, political affiliation, race sexual orientation, or social standing to intervene between my duty and my patient;
- I will maintain the utmost respect for human life from its beginning even under threat, and I will not use my medical knowledge contrary to the laws of humanity.
- I make these promises solemnly, freely and upon my honour.

Nurses and midwives also have written codes of ethics; the United Kingdom Central Council for Nursing, Midwifery and Health Visiting drew up an amendment to the 1997 Act.

Nurses, Midwives and Health Visitors (Midwives Amendment) Rules 1998

In its introduction the first points made are that:

- Midwives are accountable for their own practice in whatever environment they are practising.
- The safety and welfare of mother and baby are of primary importance.

The Rules emphasis that a practising midwife is subject to the UKCC's *Code of Professional Conduct and Midwives' Rules.*

It goes on to describe the role and activities of a midwife. These are wide-ranging and comprehensive; from the diagnosing and monitoring of normal pregnancies, providing family planning information and parenthood preparation, record keeping, and maintaining and developing competence in new skills, to the supply, possession and use of controlled drugs, as well as the administration of homeopathic or herbal substances. In the context of potential damage to the neonate during pregnancy or birth they include:

- To recognise the warning signs of abnormality in the mother or infant that necessitate referral to a doctor and to assist the latter where appropriate; also to take the necessary emergency measures in the doctor's absence.
- To examine and care for the newborn infant; to take all initiatives necessary in case of need and to carry out where necessary immediate resuscitation.
- How to deal with maternal deaths, stillbirths or neonatal death; what is required legally and how to carry through the requirements.

Advice is also about given on the importance of confidentiality and the rights of clients in relation to access to medical records.

So, both physicians and midwives have their own codes of ethics to guide them in their conduct and duty to patients; but while some clauses are quite clear in their meaning many are ambiguous and open to interpretation. The problem is that most ethical decisions are not straightforward: Most involve judgements about extremely complex situations. However, as Sim (1997) further points out, the very existence of ethical codes serves as a reminder that health care is a moral, not just a technical, enterprise.

Although ethical decisions in medicine today are central to health care practice, they are being greatly outpaced by the rapid advances in technology. Decisions now are influenced by many wide-ranging factors: socio-economic issues, legal issues, patient autonomy and rights, demographic shifts (such as the increase in the elderly population), and not least the problem of limited resources for health care in the NHS. This is why Sim feels that it is important to maintain a moral perspective that should be the foundation of any relationship and practice between doctors and patients.

MEDICAL ETHICAL DECISION MAKING

> If we want to discover the truth we must try to let our feelings be guided as much as possible by reasons, or arguments, that can be given for the opposing views. Morality is, first and foremost, a matter of consulting reason: the morally right thing to do, in any circumstance, is determined by what there are the best reasons for doing.
>
> (Rachels 1993, p.10)

Nowadays, most people are aware of and have definite views on controversial advances in biotechnology, such as human cloning, and 'designer babies'. However as Harris (1985) points out, many of our attitudes to and judgements about such problems are prompted by our deep-seated beliefs and values, which we have acquired over many years from the process of socialisation, from family upbringing and from the environment in which we live. We very rarely question them; they form part of our fundamental system of values. In medical ethics, the validity of the role of the philosopher is often questioned by those who say that health care decisions should be left in the hands of health care professionals; they are the ones who are in the clinical situation, therefore they are in the best position to decide how best to deal with medical dilemmas.

However, our feelings, views and opinions should be examined. For, as Rachels (1986) emphasises, whilst these may be a sign of 'moral seriousness' and worthy of being taken seriously, they may also serve as a barrier to our discovery of the truth. Just because we have strong feelings about an issue, this does not necessarily mean that our feelings are right. Feelings, however powerful, may not always be a reliable foundation on which to base an argument or solve a problem; they may be a result of long-standing prejudice, greed or self-interest, and cannot always be validated. It is important that we consider other points of view and evaluate both sides of an argument, basing our decisions on reason rather than feelings. Rachels (1986) believes that it is reason which distinguishes personal taste from moral judgement and illustrates his point with the following example:

If someone says, "I like coffee", that is an expression of personal taste. There is no need to defend the position, and no suggestion that everyone else should feel the same way. It does not matter either way. However, if someone claims that something is morally wrong, he does need reasons. If these reasons are sound, then others will have to acknowledge them; but if there are no good reasons for what he says then he is 'just making a noise and we need pay him no attention.' (Rachels 1986, p. 10)

Codes of medical ethics give practitioners guidelines about what is acceptable or forbidden in everyday decision-making; they also provide a basis from which discussion and reappraisal may take place when new forms of treatment are discovered. They are useful in informing the public about what kind of values and behaviour they can expect from the profession, and in setting out rules upon which disciplinary action and its implications may be instigated against any misconduct or malpractice. Conversely, they can also be a useful means of defending or supporting individuals who may challenge institutional or legal practices that they believe are against patient interests.

There are many theories of ethics, but in medical ethics, the framework for decision-making is based on two main theories and principles that are designed to help resolve some of the most difficult medical dilemmas that confront doctors and nurses. These decision-maing tools are extremely relevant in the area of midwifery and neonatal intensive care, where often decisions about treatment are not straightforward and doctors face situations where they have to choose between two equally critical or unpleasant alternatives. The decisions they reach have the potential to bring either joy and thankfulness or anguish and despair into the lives of countless families.

Hadley (2000) considers that the cost of technological advances is increasing uncertainty in medicine: this is the price we pay for progress.

In matters of life and death the onus must be on doctors to account for human factors – for anguish, for an excess of emotion – but not to allow decisions to be based only on them. The most advanced technology impoverishes us if we don't use it with a little wisdom.

(Hadley 2000, p. 42)

Ethical principles are underpinned by ethical theories, which together can provide a framework upon which difficult medical judgements can be based. The two principle theories used in medical ethics are deontology and utilitarianism.

Deontology

The word 'deontology' comes from the Greek 'deon' meaning duty. The principle is derived from the complex theories of the German philosopher Immanuel Kant (1724-1804). His ethic is based on what he called the 'categorical imperative' which takes its form in various, unchanging principles stemming from universal moral laws and emphasises one's obligation to others.

Kant's view was that duty and reason are the only rational bases for morality and that a person's action should not be motivated by feelings or emotions; only acts proceeding from goodwill are moral. So, an act which is in accordance with an individual's duty or obligation is right, and an act, which is not in accord with an individual's duty or obligation is wrong.

Kant's overriding dictum was that we are duty bound only to act on certain universal principles that any other rational person would adopt; any act by an individual must be seen and determined to be valid for everyone. In other words, when the ordinary person chooses to act in a certain way, one should always ask oneself, 'If everyone did this would it be considered good or bad?'

The principles that he felt were the basis of this universality were absolute and could not be overridden by any other principles. For example, as far as Kant was concerned it would *always* be wrong to take a life, tell a lie, steal, break a promise or leave debts unpaid, whatever the circumstances. These universal duties and laws are to be obeyed regardless of outcomes: actions themselves are important and some actions are morally necessary regardless of their consequences. Kant pointed out that sometimes the consequences of actions can be quite different from what was originally intended or anticipated; also, not everyone will always desire the same things anyway. Therefore it is futile to take the consequences into consideration: it is the *intention* of an act itself that is important, not the outcome. Consequences have no moral value in themselves.

Kant also believed that each individual has intrinsic moral worth and therefore we should respect an individual's autonomy and treat others as we would wish them to treat us. Beauchamp and Childress (1989) state that to respect the autonomy of another person is:

> To recognise that person's capacities and perspective, including his or her right to hold views, make choices and to take actions based on personal values and beliefs.
>
> (Beauchamp and Childress 1989, p. 71)

Kant also taught that if we violate someone's autonomy, by using them to fulfil our own needs and desires instead of their own, we are devaluing them and treating them merely as a means to an end. If we respect another person's autonomy, we honour their freedom to act on any decisions they have made; even if we disagree.

The problem for many who questioned Kant's absolutist views was that the approach could become too rigid and inflexible making deontology impossible in practice. One criticism was that certain actions were ruled out however much good they might achieve. For example, consider the following situation:

> A soldier is captured in wartime and interrogated about the whereabouts of his fellow officers. Should he tell the truth? Although he believes that this is always the right thing to do, he knows that by doing so he may place his comrades in mortal danger. The outcome is not certain, but it is highly likely that they too will all be captured. The problem for him is the conflict between his duty to always tell the truth and his duty of loyalty to his fellow men. Because he cannot be sure about the consequences of his actions the deontologist could be justified in replying truthfully to the enemies' questioning, for he would see it as his duty never to tell a lie. On the other hand, does he not also have a moral obligation to protect those with whom he shares a common bond of loyalty and trust?

Critics of deontology queried how it could be wrong to carry out an action that will produce the best results; surely in the example quoted above, the soldier's duty to his fellow men must outweigh his obligation to tell the truth at all times? So it appears that a number of problems could arise when the absolute deontologist tries to live out this philosophy to its full extent. Difficulties often arise if several 'duties' conflict with each other necessitating decisions about which should take precedence. How can we be sure which duties to put first, and, if there needs to be a hierarchical structure of duties, who is to decide in which order they should be placed?

For some critics, Kantian views seem to be better at determining what individuals should *not* do, than at helping them choose the right action when faced with conflicting alternatives in complicated situations. Kant's approach does not give enough weight to human intuition.

Sir William D Ross (1877–1971) offered an alternative approach to the rigid concepts of the absolute deontologist: the non-absolutist or defeasabilist view. He still believed that some actions were intrinsically right and others were wrong; for example, he felt that lying was fundamentally wrong, but that people could lie for different reasons. Some may lie from a bad motive, perhaps to cheat or defraud someone; others may lie for more noble reasons, perhaps to protect someone from harm, as in the above example.

Ross advocated that in some situations, when conflicts do arise, it is possible to distinguish between what he termed 'prima facie' duties and actual or absolute duties. He believed that there are certain moral obligations which rational human beings will accept as valid, and these will take precedence (providing there are no other conflicting moral obligations) when guiding the individual's actions. He defined these as fidelity, beneficence, non-maleficence, justice, reparation, gratitude and self-improvement.

Ross did not feel that these could be ranked in any hierarchical order, recognising that in a situation of conflict, it is the individual's duty to decide which of these prima facie duties was the most applicable when weighing the benefits and burdens. This duty would then be regarded as the absolute duty in that particular set of circumstances.

In the context of medical ethics, doctors are often faced with dilemmas that involve conflict between professional and certain other duties. The complex nature of the deontological theory of ethics is clear.

Deontology can be described as a backward-looking moral theory, concerned with concepts such as duties, rights and obligations. Right actions are those based on duty and respect for others and not based on the consequences of one's actions. The morality of an action depends on its inherent worth.

For the deontologist, it is the avoidance of wrongdoing that is important and we can achieve this by following clearly defined constraints on our behaviour. So, if we avoid telling untruths, killing or stealing, then we are acting rightly. Many might say that these views fit very well with most people's intuitive idea of what constitutes right and wrong.

Objections to deontology

Those who criticise the deontological approach believe that it is far too complicated because it shows no clear way of resolving conflicts.

Nancy Davis (1993) says that for the ordinary person compliance with rules is fairly simple. Any law abiding person will find it quite an easy matter to refrain from killing and stealing. Most people would think twice before lying under oath in a court of law. Although these are very laudable attributes, Davis points out that it is both undesirable and psychologically unsound to expect every individual to go about their lives behaving as only 'discrete rational wills' and guardians of their own virtue, unconcerned by the behaviour of others. Life is not that simple. Individuals are members of the human race and of a moral community, where interacting with others is an inevitable part of everyday life.

Life is not always about the negative (*avoiding* wrongdoing); but about positives too, like *promoting* the wellbeing of our fellow men. Davis feels that any view of morality simply as a burden imposed by external laws is too narrow and that a broader view is needed.

Utilitarianism

Whereas deontology was based on personal actions and individual integrity, utilitarianism is founded on the principle that the consequences of an action determine whether an action is right or wrong. Utilitarianism has no religious or theological basis and became popular because of its relative simplicity, avoiding the moral conflicts that can be found in deontology.

Utilitarianism originated with Jeremy Bentham (1748–1832)

who believed that 'the end justifies the means' and that basic morality is to do with maximising happiness and minimising misery. His view was that suffering is an evil and that happiness is good. So, for the utilitarian, doing the greatest good for the greatest number of people is seen as morally correct behaviour. Action should be based on usefulness: useful acts result in good and useless acts result in harm.

The utilitarian will use any means available to achieve the greater good, so personal actions are justifiable (whether they be good or bad) if performed to achieve the maximum benefit. Individuals may need to do something 'bad' in order to achieve a good result: for example, if one person's untruth means saving someone's life or stopping something awful happening, then 'the end will justify the means'.

Another proponent of the utilitarian ethic was John Stuart Mill (1806–73). He broadened the argument by proposing that an action was morally correct if it contributed to the betterment of living conditions for the majority of the people. He was therefore a fervent critic of government and institutions that did not consider the quality of life for ordinary citizens in their administrations. He was a strong advocate for social justice and individual liberty, espousing the cause of women's enfranchisement and their right to equality of educational opportunity. Utilitarianism is a forward-looking, consequentialist approach that follows no strict rules or codes. It is the outcomes of actions that determine their moral worth. In the example given previously of the soldier's dilemma about whether to tell the truth or lie to protect his friends, the utilitarian position would have no problem in justifying a lie, in order to save lives. The benefits gained by telling a lie would far outweigh the probable dreadful consequences if he told the truth and betrayed his comrades.

Objections to utilitarianism

As with deontology, there are limitations in putting this theory into practice. Some argue that trying to determine what is the 'greatest good' can be a very subjective exercise, for it is not always clear whose greatest good we are considering, or what we actually mean by 'goodness'. It is not easy to define precisely what is meant by the concepts of 'happiness' or 'goodness', so how is it then possible to use them as criteria for judgements?

Sometimes people do not agree about what they think will give them happiness, so there can be a danger of inconsistencies in decisions as a result. How does one decide who is right when conflicting views occur? Anyway, should the maximisation of happiness necessarily be the only overriding moral principle?

Another problem for the utilitarian is that the ordinary moral principles of respect for the individual's autonomy, honesty and justice may be overridden if the general happiness of the group, or society in general, requires it.

Also, is it really true that it is always the *consequences* of actions that matter, or can some actions in themselves be bad? For example, would it be considered moral to commit horrific atrocities in order to achieve a greater good eventually?

Another problem is that it is not always possible to judge for certain what the long-term outcomes of an action will be. Therefore for some people, attempting to judge consequences is irrelevant.

In order to address some of these issues, Rule Utilitarianism emerged; this states that the welfare of society in general is important. Therefore society must, by the best means available, produce rules and laws which will give maximum benefit to the maximum number of people, so that individuals within society know where their rights and responsibilities lie. These modified theories of utilitarianism have accepted the view that certain actions, such as lying and cheating, are intrinsically wrong, even when the consequences are not bad. In the same way, many deontologists accept the idea that it is rare for consequences not to be considered whenever actions are taken. Thus the two theories begin to merge.

Translating theory into practice

Pritchard (1996) describes these differing theories as 'silk screens' that are placed over the facts. If one looks at the same facts from differing standpoints (i.e. different philosophical theories), it will be possible to come up with two opposite actions to produce a good solution. Viewing a problem through the screen of utilitarianism would generate a solution that would produce the greatest good for the largest number of people. The same problem, viewed through the screen of deontology, would produce a very different solution. In this case, the professional would regard their duty to the patient as paramount, irrespective of any other competing needs or consequences. Deontologists may also question whether, on the whole, it would be better to aim for doing the least harm for all rather than producing the greatest amount of good, particularly in the field of medical care.

Theories and principles are fine if one is merely hypothesising about a problem, but as Jonathan Moreno (1999) points out, this is the difference between moral philosophers and the medical staff who are expected to make decisions in a real-life clinical situation. 'Detachment should remain at the heart of what it is about, but in a clinical context it is a plan of action that is needed.' Moreno reminds us again that in a pluralistic society, when there are so many moral points of view that differ, there can never be any easy answers.

Many believe that professional ethics for the medical profession is particularly suited to the deontological approach. Within this system individuals can be allotted specific roles and duties. Nevertheless, difficulties for many doctors and nurses may arise when conflicts of duties occur in a number of ways; sometimes clashes between their values and beliefs as an individual member of society and their duty as a practitioner can be a source of tension. Interpretation of these principles is often an individual matter, so, for example, doctors who have strong opinions against abortion on the grounds that it is morally wrong under any circumstances, will find it hard to advise women who request termination for social or economic reasons. Often, they will pass the patient over to a colleague who they know will be more sympathetic to the appeal; thus they avoid any conflict with their conscience. The deontological view would be that the doctor has acted in accordance with his own conscience and therefore it is up to other practitioners to do the same. The utilitarian would have less difficulty in agreeing to the request, for they could argue that although abortion may not a desirable act in itself, if the outcome helped the woman and her family to cope better with life, then 'the end would justify the means'.

Nowadays, conflict can also be seen in the way many doctors are reacting to government policy about hospital management and patient care, believing that hospital trusts are more concerned with utilitarian targets (that involve assessments of financial criteria and cost benefits) than with quality care for individual patients.

Another source of variance can arise when a doctor's professional loyalty to colleagues is seen to conflicy with their duty of care to patients. We have seen that, although the Hippocratic Oath had loyalty to one's colleagues as the first principle, the Declaration of Geneva, made it clear that the doctor's first allegiance was to his patient. Despite this, the close bond of fellowship within the profession is very difficult to break. Over the past few years, cases of horrendous practice have been brought to court; the doctors involved may have been known in the profession for their cavalier approach to patients, but none of their colleagues could find it within themselves to 'blow the whistle'.

The ethicist's role is to help find new ways to guide these rival belief systems into workable practices. This entails being familiar with the fundamental practices within the health care system, understanding the nuances of language and political structures and the processes of hospital care and management, and being involved with decisions relating to real situations and particular cases (Moreno, 1999).

PRINCIPLES USED IN MEDICAL ETHICS

> An ethical principle can be regarded as the statement of fundamental ethical value or belief, which grounds and justifies specific ethical decisions and actions.
>
> (Julius Sim 1997, p. 15)

The four principles which have been widely accepted as a basis for ethical decision-making in British medical practice are:

- Beneficence
- Non-maleficence
- Respect for autonomy
- Justice.

These are the basic precepts from which doctors make their clinical decisions in all branches of medicine. In the field of neonatal care, the question of what kind of treatment should be given to the very immature and sick premature baby is underpinned by principles which include preservation of life, alleviation of suffering, non-maleficence, patient autonomy and justice.

According to Tyson (1995) 'when ethical problems arise in the care of these infants, there is usually conflict between two or more of these principles. How best to address the conflict between these abstract principles while dealing with the concrete problem of very premature babies has been debated for years'.

Beneficence and non-maleficence

Some ethicists would argue that these two principles cannot be considered separately as they are two aspects of the same code and both fundamental to the Hippocratic Oath, which states:

> I will use treatment to help the sick according to my ability and my judgement, but will never use it to injure or wrong them.
> (Singleton and McLaren 1995, p. 40)

The principle of beneficence says that one should endeavour to promote the interests and wellbeing of others by conferring benefits on them. A beneficent act is intended to maximise another's best interests and Sim (1997) sees it as taking one of two forms:

- A person may act to produce a positive good for someone, or
- A person may act to remove someone from harm.

To do something positive, like giving someone food or making them comfortable when they are ill, would be an example of the first sort; stopping a child from running across a busy street and certain injury would illustrate the second.

Most doctors, as Gillon (1985) points out, do place the interests of patients before their own and are also expected by society to have a duty of beneficence, to do their best for all the sick, but particularly those who are their patients. He does however caution that certain constraints accompany beneficence:

- The need to respect the *autonomy* of those who are to be helped. It is important to discover what they actually want – not what we think they should want.
- The need to ensure that any help is not given at too high a price, so that the duty of beneficence is always tempered by the duty of *non-maleficence*.
- The duty of beneficence needs to be tempered by the duty of *justice*, for the needs of the individual should be considered in relation to the rights and needs of others in society.

Gillon also feels that beneficence refers to subtler and less quantifiable requirements of the doctor-patient relationship. These include effective, adequate and sympathetic communication, and a friendly and open approach between the practitioner and the patient.

The principle of non-maleficence ('*primum non nocere*; above all... do no harm') refers to the idea that one ought to do no harm to another person, and that a morally correct action should never promote harm, pain or suffering.

However, as Sim (1997) further points out, while beneficence and non-maleficence seem to be similar in position, they approach from a different standpoint. Beneficence can be seen as a *positive* requirement to help others; non-maleficence is more of a negative requirement, in that it imposes restraints on any actions that might harm others.

The principle of non-maleficence is often considered to take precedence over beneficence in medical ethics, because in health care the deontological approach is usually adopted and is fundamental to the promises enshrined within the Hippocratic Oath. The *absolute* deontologist will see their primary obligation as doing no harm to anyone, which is greater than their duty to offer benefit; however, the *defeasabilist* deontologist would deal with any conflict of duties arising in a particular case, by considering what their *prima facie* duty should be and acting accordingly.

However Beauchamp and Childress (1989) challenge this view, arguing that the principle of beneficence (that is, promoting the welfare of patients, not just avoiding harm) should be the goal of health care. The utilitarian approach would be do as much good as possible. Maximising benefits is important and sometimes an initially bad action may be justified eventually because more people gain as a result. In a medical situation this could mean that a temporary harm to a patient, in the short term, may actually produce greater benefits in the long term, not only to that patient, but also to many more in the future.

In the field of neonatal care, this could be a potential problem. Both Miller (1996) and Mitchell (1986) hint that some pioneering doctors in this area may allow their enthusiasm for improving techniques to actually outweigh the possible suffering caused to the individual infant in the process. This fervour can sometimes be triggered not only by the need to benefit other babies in the long term, but sometimes by a doctor's own desire to be first in the field to save the smallest or the youngest baby. If this is the reason for their actions, such doctors are certainly guilty of putting their own interests before those of their patients, and in the process endangering both principles of beneficence and non-maleficence.

In this sort of situation, some might question whether doctors have the right to subject these tiny infants to the stress and pain involved in aggressive therapies, knowing that they might die or suffer severe impairment as a result. Is the individual baby paying too high a price for the benefit of others in society (or for the professional ambition of an over-zealous doctor)? The problem seems to be that it is almost impossible to estimate how much pain a premature baby is suffering. The general practice is to keep them heavily sedated on morphine in the first few days, so it can be assumed that they feel relatively comfortable. But the fine line between heavy sedation and allowing the child to waken enough to begin to breathe unaided is very tenuous. When this stage is reached it becomes more difficult to get the balance right and pain management is more difficult. One has to ask whether the treatment is doing more harm than good.

Some would have no doubt that it is unethical to expose the individual infant to pain and suffering, even though future children could benefit from the action. The deontologist would see the practice as abhorrent, for their duty would be to inflict no harm on another person; any future benefits to that child or any other would have no relevance to their argument. For them, the action itself is important, not the outcome.

Others, like Wells (1989), in accepting that the two principles need to be weighed together when making medical judgements, take the utilitarian view that harm may necessary in order to achieve good; they therefore support the view that experimental treatment on a premature baby would be acceptable if, in the long term, it will be of benefit to many more babies.

It goes without saying that without neonatal intensive care, most, if not all, very premature babies would die within a few minutes, hours or days after birth. But, writes Tyson (1995), it is possible for neonatal intensive care to make the outcome worse by prolonging death and causing intense suffering at the same time. Some parents view this 'care', along with the probability of facing a lifetime suffering extensive neurological damage, as worse than death for their baby. So it could be argued that it is not always beneficial for babies to be saved, irrespective of their gestational age or condition, and that treatment may therefore be difficult to justify in ethical terms. Aggressive treatments to prolong the life of a very premature infant have the potential to cause severe suffering both at the time and in future, and need to be carefully considered and justified. Views about what constitutes harm can have a fundamental effect on what course of action to take. One doctor or parent may see death as the ultimate harm to the child, while another might view death as a benefit and a release from suffering. Different views about what constitutes harm can be a source of conflict between practitioners and parents.

Respect for autonomy

This principle refers to the right to make one's own decisions and to be self governing, providing that this right does not impinge on the rights of others.

In the field of medical ethics, respect for the patient's autonomy has become an important consideration; it is an integral part of deontological theory. Of course, to be autonomous, the patient must be competent to make informed decisions when consenting to treatment. A competent patient has the right to refuse medical treatment on any grounds, even when doctors consider refusal to be against their best interests.

The principle of autonomy will override both principles of beneficence and non-maleficence, providing the individual has been fully informed about their condition and what available alternatives there may be for treatment; and very crucially, providing that they are competent to decide what is in their own best interests.

> The starting point for consent is actually competence.
>
> (Draper 1996, p. 24)

Anyone who is incompetent cannot be autonomous. Being autonomous means that individuals are competent to make informed choices about their lives; they are in a position to decide whether to accept or ignore advice given by another person, even if that person is an expert and has warned of the dangers of ignoring his/her advice.

However, as Draper (1996) further points out, competence may not be an absolute state. Some people may be competent to make some decisions, but other issues may prove too intricate.

Individuals may be competent to handle difficult choices on some occasions, but not others; for example, decisions made under extreme pressure or at a point in one's life when things look bleak can often be regretted later, when we are seeing things from a different perspective.

Children may not always be incompetent, neither may people with learning disabilities. They may be able to make certain judgements, providing the various complexities have been suitably explained to them.

Singleton and McLaren (1995) draw our attention to the important concept of the 'future autonomy' of the child. They make the point that only if there is a possibility that the child might have decision-making capacities in the future, does the principle of autonomy become relevant.

Here we are discussing issues around saving the lives of marginally viable newborn babies, who cannot be consulted, as autonomous individuals. They may never be able to make any decisions, informed or otherwise. They are in no position to value their own life now, and may never develop the intellectual faculties to be aware of themselves as individuals in the future either. In the eyes of the law they are incompetent and unable to make decisions regarding their future. This raises the question of whether the principle of autonomy has any moral bearing on the decisions about the treatment of these babies.

One of the vital points to consider here is the fact that not all of the babies whose lives are saved by invasive technology will grow up with massive damage; some will have more moderate degrees of special need. We need to recognise that the principle of autonomy is very closely linked to the principle of justice and that the rights and dignity of these people are often ignored or overruled, because of the lack of resources to help them in achieving their goals.

Harris (1985) and Glover (1997), would argue that any young baby, whether disabled or not, has not yet reached the stage of being a real 'person' who can form and express their own preferences. So the principle of autonomy is irrelevant not just to premature babies with profound mental and physical impairment, but to any infant. However, Hayry (1998) makes an interesting point about the ability of human infants to make their feelings known in certain situations. She describes a hypothetical situation where a child may be deprived of food and drink for a given length of time to see how it would react. Obviously she is not advocating this as a real experiment, but she indicates that the wishes or will of the infant would be implied by its behaviour. It seems fairly certain that the child would cry, or show other signs of dehydration or distress by which we could deduce that they were unhappy with their treatment, even though they could not articulate their feelings.

Some argue that the parents are the best people to decide what is best for their offspring. Mitchell (1986) quotes an American study that issued guidelines to the effect that parents are the best people to take on the responsibility, providing they are themselves competent, that both are in agreement about the treatment plan, and more importantly, that their principle concern is to act in the child's best interests. Others would disagree, challenging the idea of parental autonomy on the grounds that the parents may not be in a position to know exactly what those best interests are. Parents do not always have the necessary knowledge to fully understand the complex nature of medical problems, and it is unfair to expect them to make decisions when they themselves are suffering the shock of the premature birth and the trauma of seeing their baby in intensive care. All these factors may have a profound influence on any rational choices they make about further treatment. In these circumstances, it could be argued that the medical team should have the major input when deciding what to do next.

Tyson (1995) points out that, in the end, we do have to leave these decisions in the hands of parents and health professionals on behalf of the child, but emphasises that decisions about withdrawing or withholding treatment for the very premature infant involves weighing the same fundamental ethical considerations as would be faced whether the patient was five days, five months or fifty years old.

Paternalism

There is another principle that needs to be examined, that may conflict with the principle of patient autonomy. Paternalism has its roots in the idea of a caring parent, someone who makes decisions on behalf of another, in the belief that they are acting in the best interest of that person, just as a caring parent sometimes needs to take decisions to protect a child who is too young to know the pitfalls or dangers of a situation. The child may not like or see the reason for the decision at the time, but the parent believes that, given time, his offspring will appreciate the wisdom of the action. In the past, it was often the case that patients always bowed to the judgement of their doctors; patient autonomy was not an issue and the paternalistic approach adopted by the medical profession was accepted as always being in the patient's best interests. In essence, paternalism is benevolent in intention.

As Gillon (1985) points out, the Hippocratic Oath says nothing about seeking the wishes of the patient, or explaining the likely outcomes of any form of treatment. Its basic assumption seems to be that the doctor, by virtue of his expertise, knows what is best for the patient. A doctor who practices paternalism ignores their patients' capacity to make their own decisions and the patient plays a passive role in receiving health care.

Some patients are more than happy to allow their doctor to make decisions for them. Some may wish their doctor to shield them from any unpalatable or distressing revelations about their true state of health. Indeed, as Singleton and McLaren (1995) point out, there are situations when decision making on behalf of a patient is not only morally acceptable, but necessary. For example, in an emergency situation, when action needs to be taken fast to save a life, there may not be time to explain the nature of the treatment until the crisis is over.

Nevertheless, if a practitioner is overly paternalistic in his attitude to normal patient care, he may compromise a patient's autonomy, override their express wishes or not even bother to ask their opinion. He may also restrict the choices by offering biased or selective alternatives when giving information about different types of available treatment; or by being less than frank about a patient's true condition. If a prognosis is poor, he may not reveal the truth, in the belief that he is protecting the patient from worry. Sometimes, although the patient may be kept in the dark about the truth of his condition, the closest relatives may be given the bad news instead. This in itself often leads to tension and conflict within the family at a time when emotions are already running high.

Some doctors may defend these courses of action by arguing that, ethically, they are simply putting the principles of beneficence or non-maleficence before that of patient autonomy. They could say that patients are not medically qualified to make informed decisions about their condition and cannot understand the intricacies of the recommended treatment. Therefore the doctor is in the best position to know what is truly in the best interests of his patient. Just as a parent sometimes needs to act against their child's wishes, for the good of that child, a doctor may feel the need to ignore or override the patient's wishes in order to do his best for them in the long term.

However, as Gillon (1985) further points out, it does not automatically follow that the patient will suffer less, or worry less, if someone else is making the decisions, omitting to tell them the truth or giving biased information about treatments. Also, when patients' relatives need to keep secrets from their loved ones, when prognoses are bad, this can put a tremendous strain on family relationships at a time when stress levels are already high. Then, if the truth eventually comes out, it can cause further distress to all concerned, in addition to a loss of confidence in the doctor-patient relationship.

The move towards patient autonomy has arisen because questions were beginning to be asked about whether doctors were any more qualified to make moral decisions about someone else's life than anyone else. Are they really in the best position to know whether the decisions they take will always be of real benefit to that patient?

This becomes very relevant in the case of the very premature infant, a newborn whose prognosis is so poor and future so bleak that they will always have to rely on others for their every need. Surely in this situation the doctor is in no better a position to make the ethical decisions about its future than the parents, who will ultimately have responsibility for the child.

There will be further discussion about the important subjects of paternalism and autonomy in Section 4 which considers the dilemmas facing doctors and parents about whether to withhold or withdraw treatment for the very ill neonate.

Justice

In medical ethics the principles of beneficence, non-maleficence and autonomy are all concerned with the care of the individual. The principle of justice is not only concerned with the individual but is used within the wider context, to consider fair and morally acceptable ways of distributing resources within society. At the macro level it is applied when governments and local authorities decide where to place their priorities when it is time to allocate their annual funding. At the micro level it is concerned with the distribution of benefits to individual patients; who gets what treatment, when and why? Within the health care budget there are many competing claims on funds; how much should be spent on different hospitals, treatments and technology. In the narrower framework of neonatal care, questions are prompted about whether it is right to spend large amounts of the budget on providing expensive technology and resources in neonatal intensive care, which will benefit a few high risk babies; or whether it is better to help more babies who are less likely to have severe disabilities. In the wider context, it is important to see how these decisions have a 'knock on' effect on the way resources are allocated to those very premature babies who were saved but have grown up with severe mental and physical disabilities, and their families.

The final section of this book considers the various theories of distributive justice and their application to the treatment of very premature babies in neonatal units, their families, and children and adults with very special needs.

PART 3

The sanctity of life

Part 3 considers the concept of the sanctity of life, and highlights an ethical dilemma concerning the concept of personhood.

PART CONTENTS

8

The value of life

> Of the ethical and moral questions before doctors today, the most divisive revolve around matters of life and death and the concept of the sanctity of human life.
>
> (Brazier 1987, p. 20)

> Few moral convictions are more deeply ingrained than that of the sanctity of life.
>
> (Kuhse 1987, p. 2)

With the increasing sophistication of medical technology and practice, the boundaries between life and death are becoming less clear. Doctors are gaining more and more control over machinery which can preserve life or end it.

Traditionally, the phrase 'sanctity of life' has deep roots in the religious philosophy of most world faiths, and religion and medicine have been interrelated for many centuries. In fact, in ancient times the role of priest and physician were interchangeable. So it is necessary first of all to examine the concept, to clarify what we mean by the term, and to consider the implications.

Different cultures view the concept in different ways. Morrison and Demichele (1997) write that doctors are not always aware of the beliefs held by patients about their religious obligations with regard to their treatment. They emphasise the importance of understanding cultural differences when decisions about life and death are being considered:

> For physicians, nurses and social workers to understand the motivations and beliefs driving a dying patient's thinking, they must understand their own beliefs, which is even more of a challenge.
> (Morrison and Demichele 1997, p. 72)

If patients (or families) view life from a religious perspective, then they may accept unfavourable events, even death itself, with composure and equanimity, believing them to be ordained by the will of God. One of the roles of religious belief is to lift human beings and equip them with a faith to overcome pain and death.

However, as society becomes more secularised there is a growing movement to explore further, to find a more acceptable ethic that does not rely on a belief in God. For many people, the theological arguments for the sanctity of life lack consistency and clarity, and as we shall see, the phrase can mean different things to different people.

In the context of the doctor-patient relationship, cultural differences need to be acknowledged and respected. This chapter examines the sanctity of life doctrine from an Eastern (Buddhist and Hindu) perspective, from a Western (Judeo-Christian) perspective, and from a secular point of view.

EASTERN TRADITIONS

Morrison and Demichele (1997) point out that in the Asian tradition, boundaries between the self and others are less rigidly drawn than in the West. The whole of life is interconnected, so that there is more sense of mutual obligation. Every individual has a responsibility towards family and others in the community and they have a more indirect and sensitive approach in interpersonal communication. In addition, there is a great emphasis placed on hierarchical structures in society and family life; great respect is given to education and career prospects. The combination of these attitudes means that communication between doctor and patient or patient's family may be somewhat inhibited.

Death itself is viewed as part of the cycle of life, but even though patient and family are aware that the end is near, in many situations nothing is mentioned and discussion with doctors is closed down.

Hinduism

The Hindu word for 'God' is Brahman, and the Hindu faith is based on a belief in Brahman who is the creator and great truth behind all things in the universe. As humans we are permeated by a spirit which is called the 'atman' and the aim in this life is to unite the atman within ourselves with the universal spirit of Brahman the creator, through meditation and good living.

The Hindu believes in the law of karma (or cause and effect) and reincarnation, so that how we behave in this life affects the conditions we have to face in our next life. Because of our imperfections as human beings, it may take us many lifetimes of service and meditation to learn all the lessons we need, to achieve perfection when the atman and Brahman are united. In this context, death is not to be feared and it is important for the Hindu to experience a 'good death', which means to accept it calmly and to be in control. Morrison and Demichele (1997) point out that for the Hindu, living is more than being alive. Quality of life plays a large part in the way a Hindu views the definition of life and death. The relationship between mind and body is so important, that the Hindu would uphold the view that because pain and suffering could interfere with the process of a good death, then the administration of drugs which will ease pain but are also likely to shorten the patient's life is acceptable, if the patient feels that the body is becoming a burden and a hindrance to the progress of the spirit. Pain and suffering may interfere with the composure and concentration of the mind at the point of death and therefore impede progress into the next incarnation. On the other hand, the Hindu tradition is opposed to active euthanasia, believing it to be a form of suicide that will affect the next life after reincarnation. For by deliberately cutting short this life (his Karma), he is destined to carry it with him into the next reincarnation.

Buddhism

This philosophy stemmed from Hinduism and so shares its roots and some of its philosophy. The Buddhist holds a more agnostic view about the existence of a universal creator, but firmly believes in the law of Karma; that what we sow, we reap in the next life. The difference is that Buddhism teaches that we alone are responsible for our actions and as long as we do as much good as we can here and now, then the reward will be in our next incarnation. Each reincarnation is a progression and the aim is to escape more rebirths by attaining 'Nirvana', a state of perfection achieved through meditation. It is a state of mind, which will free the Buddhist from materialism and all the accompanying negative thoughts and emotions, like greed and envy. Many believe that Nirvana is the equivalent of the Christian concept of Heaven, but in fact, it differs in a fundamental way: Nirvana can be experienced in this life, in the here and now, whereas the idea of Heaven is always a future promise of being with God in the life after death. The Buddhist principle of 'ahimsa' (non harming) leads the follower to respect all forms of life, drawing no moral distinction between different forms of life. They believe that every life, whether it is human or non-human, has intrinsic value and therefore is entitled to full moral respect from the time of conception till death. As we humans have all emerged from some primitive life form through many rebirths, all creation deserves respect. So there would be no moral difference between the harming of a tiny insect and harming a human being. The Buddhist believes that everything in the whole of nature is interconnected. If we harm one part, it will have repercussions elsewhere; therefore it is imperative that we try to live in harmony with all creation.

As with the Hindu, the state of mind at the point of death is important for the Buddhist. Their aim is to achieve a state of calm and composure, and relatives may wish to help them achieve this by chanting or meditating around the dying patient. They often refuse the use of drugs or any medication that may dull the senses at this time, so that the mind remains as clear as possible right to the end. Only in extreme suffering will the Buddhist accept pain relief, and even then only if it does not affect their clarity of mind.

JUDEO-CHRISTIAN PERSPECTIVE

According to Mason and McCall Smith (1999) the Judeo-Christian ethic has had a profound impact on Western thought and continues to influence contemporary debate about the sanctity of life.

People often say that life is sacred. They almost never mean what they say. They do not mean, as their words seem to imply, that life itself is sacred ... When people say that life is sacred, it is human life they have in mind.

(Singer 1996, p. 72)

Although the tradition teaches that life is a gift from God and is therefore sacred, there is a distinction between human life and that of other species. Here, the doctrine teaches that man was made in the image of God and has therefore more intrinsic value than any other animal life form, because he is the pinnacle of all creation.

Judaism

The teachings of Judaism are committed to the sanctity of life doctrine and the foundation for this belief lies in the Old Testament creation stories found in the book of Genesis. Because of his unique position in relation to God, Man also has power over all other living things, whether plant or animal and can use them for his own needs.

Then God said "And now we will make human beings; they will be like us and resemble us. They will have power over the fish, the birds and all animals, domestic and wild, large and small."

(Genesis 1 v.26 Good News Bible)

God is the giver of life; therefore only God is permitted to take it away.

Morrison and Demichele (1997) tell us that Jewish faith today emphasises the individual's obligations and responsibility to God. The Torah is the main reference point of authority for all Jews, including the doctor. In fact, orthodox Jewish physicians have a 'divine obligation' to treat patients with every available means to preserve the sanctity of life. For the Jew, self-determination and autonomy are inappropriate concepts; family and community are the most important criteria.

Some orthodox theologians teach that there is always a hope and possibility of recovery, even from potentially fatal diseases, and therefore discontinuing treatment is wrong; so the orthodox Jewish patient is obliged to accept all medication or treatment that will preserve life for as long as possible until they are 'very near' death.

Orthodox Jews do not accept that brain death is an acceptable definition of death, so, for them, to remove a patient from life support is as good as murdering him. However there are others, for example Conservative and Reform Jews, who support a more secular approach to the sanctity of life doctrine. Their view is that withdrawal of life support should be permitted where there is no meaningful hope of recovery.

In all sections of Judaism, euthanasia and suicide are strictly forbidden.

Christianity

Jesus himself was a Jew and steeped in Old Testament philosophy. Despite this, he is said to have challenged the Jewish law on many occasions, but his teachings always uphold the Jewish views about the sanctity of human life and man's special relationship with God.

The ethics of Jesus were based on his new commandment: 'As I have loved you, you are to love one another.' He taught respect for individuals. His whole ministry was geared to the care and needs of the weakest in society, including those with mental and physical disabilities. There are also frequent references to Jesus' attitude to children in the Bible; he often held them up as an example of how we, as adults, should aim to be. His teaching was against the exploitation and suffering of the most vulnerable groups in society. So the traditional Christian ethic is to do with valuing individuals for their intrinsic worth, whether they are able bodied or multiply handicapped, regardless of any real or potential value to society.

In addition, belief in the resurrection is central to Christian teaching; this gives Christians an extra spiritual dimension to life, which links them to the creator with whom they will be reunited in death. Christians believe that all human beings possess an immortal soul that, in essence, is the true self. For the Christian, death is viewed as the beginning of a new existence, with God, for all eternity. Because life is God given, it follows that only God can take it away; therefore, killing another person or even killing oneself is against the divine law. This leads to strong views in relation to the practice of abortion and euthanasia and is particularly strong in Roman Catholic teaching. This is evidenced by the words of Archbishop Murphy O'Connor during the court case Re A (the case of the conjoined twins):

Human life is sacred, that is inviolable, so that one should never aim to cause an innocent person's death by act or omission.

The problem for the Christian tradition is that different denominations have differing views on exactly how they interpret the doctrine.

The Roman Catholic Church forbids abortion even in circumstances where continuing the pregnancy may mean the death of the mother; but it has formulated doctrines to accommodate certain problematic areas where the sanctity of life doctrine is endangered. The doctrine of double effect and the doctrine of acts and omissions are in place to help in grey areas where 'cut and dried' decisions are impossible.

The Protestant churches and the Jewish faith do approve abortion in certain circumstances: to save the life of the mother or to abort an abnormal foetus, or in the case of pregnancy resulting from rape. In either case the life of the mother is given preference over the life of the unborn child.

David Keown (1995) tells us that the Anglican and Catholic bishops' joint view (1993) on this point of medical ethics states:

- All human beings are to be valued, irrespective of age, sex, religion, social status or their potential achievement. (para. 3)
- The deliberate taking of a human life is prohibited, except in self defence or the legitimate defence of others. (para.13)

In the case of euthanasia, again different denominations have differing approaches. The 1980 Roman Catholic Declaration on Euthanasia forbids any treatment that will deliberately end life; however, extraordinary means need not be used in order simply to maintain life. Some Catholic theologians believe that a patient's willingness to forego further treatment indicates recognition of his mortality and failing condition, with a reluctance to use valuable resources that will be of more benefit to others. These unselfish acts will lead to spiritual growth: the acceptance of suffering brings the individual nearer to Christ. This is important particularly if life is nearing its end. Discouraging the use of analgesics also aids spiritual progress; clarity of mind is essential for the important act of confession.

This approach is questioned by others in the Catholic tradition, who say that if a patient is in need of pain-killing drugs and requests them, they should be administered, even though they may impair respiratory function and reduce consciousness.

Some sections of the Protestant tradition oppose both active and passive euthanasia; others, while rejecting the notion of active euthanasia, are more sympathetic to the idea of passive euthanasia. Many denominations accept the practice of withdrawing life support from people when death is inevitable, favouring the view that it is preferable to allow the patient to 'die with dignity'. They teach that an individual may refuse treatment if the measures proposed serve only to extend the dying process.

Only the Methodist Church has stated that there may be certain circumstances when active euthanasia can be morally justifiable.

It seems that despite the theological differences about which kinds of life have value, both Eastern and Western traditions share the view that all human life has intrinsic value and therefore deserves respect. Nevertheless there is also the counter view that human life need not be preserved at all costs. These paradoxes have led some to question the validity of this claim of various religions to uphold the sanctity of life principle. If all human life is of equal value, irrespective of its condition, then why is it that the life of a mother is seen to be more valuable than the life of her unborn child? Why is it deemed permissible to sanction the withdrawal of artificial life support for a multiply disabled newborn?

Hostler (1988) argues that theological arguments are inconsistent and a weak defence for the sanctity of life principle. He sees the concept of immortality of the soul as weakening the sanctity of life view: if the soul is immortal and represents the true self, then to kill the physical body is not to do actual harm to that person, but in effect, will free them from their earthly body and allow their soul to unite with the eternal, which is in fact their ultimate aim. Therefore, Hostler maintains that the theological arguments against the killing of another human being seem to hinge upon the idea that such killing is an act against God, rather than a harm to the person concerned. Kuhse (1987) agrees that following such an argument, one could conclude that it is not human life itself that is inviolable or has sanctity, but the will of God.

Kuhse further points out that the sanctity of life doctrine is not always against killing: while it is generally believed by most people that killing is wrong, there are wide discrepancies in deciding whether it is wrong in all circumstances, or whether it can sometimes be justified. Even in theological doctrines there is no imperative to regard human life as sacrosanct. For example, to kill in self-defence or in a 'just' war situation is not seen as morally wrong. Therefore it must be the intentional taking of innocent lives that is wrong.

Within the Hippocratic Oath, the patient is under the protection of the doctor and therefore the 'innocent party'. However, as Mason and McCall Smith (1999) state, neither the Hippocratic Oath nor the Declaration of Geneva states that doctors are obliged always to provide treatment. The emphasis is on 'non-maleficence' and the phrase 'do no harm' leads to a more pragmatic approach, that can be open to interpretation.

In view of the fact that society has become more secularised in the past few decades, many now believe that it is time to explore a more secular argument for the sanctity of life principle.

> Few moral convictions are more deeply ingrained than that of the sanctity of life. However, if plausible once, the view that life is a divine gift (bestowed, sustained, and finally reclaimed by God) is now more difficult to maintain.
>
> (Helga Kuhse 1987, p. 2)

So, what arguments can be submitted in support of the secular stance? And if the sanctity of life argument is abandoned, are we acknowledging that killing is not intrinsically wrong? If this is the case then where could these arguments lead?

TOWARDS A SECULAR VIEW

> Once challenged, the traditional ethic crumples. Weakened by the decline in religious authority and the rise of a better understanding of the origins and nature of our species, that ethic is now being brought undone by changes in medical technology with which its inflexible structures cannot cope.
>
> (Peter Singer 1994, p. 4)

Brazier (1992) believes that there is a secular basis on which the sanctity of life doctrine can be argued, for both atheists and agnostics share the view that taking life is unacceptable. There is a deep human instinct that to kill another human being is intrinsically wrong because life is the individual's precious possession and 'all other possessions, all potential joys, depend upon his continual existence'. A threat to an individual's right to life can have repercussions for the whole of society and threatens the principle of autonomy.

However even though this may be the case, even though most people believe that life is sacred and that to kill someone is wrong, there are wide discrepancies in deciding whether it is wrong in *all* circumstances. Can killing another person sometimes be justified?

Dworkin (1993) argues the view that life can be seen as important and valuable in itself, irrespective of any other considerations such as its quality or usefulness to others. He feels that our lives contain many examples of our valuing objects or events for their own sakes rather than for any utilitarian purpose. Some areas of knowledge, nature and art may be considered valuable in themselves, and people will go to great lengths to preserve and protect them, because of their inherent qualities rather than any instrumental value they may have. Further, Dworkin cites a general concern for the preservation of endangered species, noting a general respect for the natural process of evolution and the abhorrence that most people feel towards wanton acts of destruction and violation of the natural world. The sense that we should respect the processes of life and not act to harm them is irrespective of any religious or secular view and is shared by most rational human beings.

> Something is sacred or inviolable when its deliberate destruction would dishonour what ought to be honoured.
>
> (Richard Dworkin 1993, p. 74)

If all the previously mentioned things have intrinsic value and deserve our respect, then human life, the highest form of natural creation, cannot be excluded from the argument.

Heifetz (1996) agrees that the principle serves to uphold a respect for life and helps to counter the dangers of becoming too mechanical or impersonal when decisions about human life are considered. He cites this deeply ingrained concept that life is worth preserving and our natural instincts to protect and nurture our offspring. Heifetz believes that public attitudes are deeply affected by what we feel about our own offspring: this is why there is such fierce disagreement in the debate about the sanctity of life for the very ill neonate.

What makes human life valuable?

"Jodie did not learn to sit or crawl, or bat toys, or even reach towards sounds. He changed so little that I stopped believing in development. I

> thought he would cry forever. I wondered whether his life held any chance of happiness. I wondered whether it was worth living." Jodie was severely brain damaged, suffered from hydrocephalus and was blind.
>
> (Featherstone 1980, p. 5)

If, as Glover suggests, some human lives are not worth living, how are we to make that judgement? By what criteria do we begin to assess the value of life?

John Harris (1985) states that equality before the law and equal entitlement to the care and protection of the state (which includes medical care) are basic human rights. Each of us is entitled to the same care, respect and protection as anyone else. He explains:

> We are interested in why and whether people have a particular significance and value simply because they are people and have whatever it takes to be a person, and are not quite different sorts of beings, animals or plants perhaps, which do not have what it takes.
>
> (Harris 1985, p. 8)

Harris tries to identify morally relevant features that allow us to respect and value ourselves and others, but also distinguish us from plants or other animal life forms. Harris and Glover (1977) agree that to try to itemise all the criteria of a life worth living is an impossible task; what is of value to one person can be of little value to another. Harris (1985) feels that we should not judge the value of life in quantitative terms, but rather on the basis of whether the individuals concerned have the capacity to give an account, or value their own life. We do not need to know the reasons why life is valuable, only that the individuals do value their own lives. An act that deliberately ends a life is wrong, if it deprives that person of this capacity to value his or her own life. For Harris, it is not just self-awareness that is a major criterion for the value of life, but the notion that the individual must be aware that they have a life to value; that they have a concept of knowing that they exist in time (that is, in the past, the present and the future). Otherwise, they would have no view about whether they wished to live or not.

Of course, following this line of argument one could ask: 'If a person does not value their own life, then it would not be wrong for them to kill themselves, or for anyone else to help them in the act if that was their wish?'

Rachels (1986) puts the concept differently, by contrasting being alive in a biological sense as opposed to being alive in a biographical sense, and in this context sums up the difference between a person and a mere human being. What gives life value and meaning is the sum of one's aspirations, decisions, activities, projects and human relationships; in other words, being alive in a 'biographical' sense.

This is similar to Singer's (1996) view of personhood and is summed up by Singleton and McLaren (1995):

> Although it is necessary to be alive in the biological sense in order to have a biographical life, the former is not sufficient for a biographical life.
>
> (Singleton and McLaren 1995, p. 700)

Are some lives more valuable than others?

An unqualified belief in the sanctity of life means that every life has intrinsic value, regardless of its present condition, prognosis or future quality of life. However, both Singer (1996) and Glover (1977) dispute this. The very people who advocate the principle, whether it is in law or theology, will also accept that it is acceptable practice not to try and save a very severely malformed baby, or to allow someone to die who has advanced Alzheimer's disease, or to withdraw food and water from a patient in a persistent vegetative state. As Glover (1977) points out, if every life does have equal value, then it should follow that morally there is no difference between the states of being conscious or unconscious. He argues that most people who would uphold the sanctity of life principle, would also accept that being alive is only of instrumental value and it is actually consciousness that is intrinsically valuable. Singer (1996) adds to this by proposing that in the light of new invasive technology, the law does acknowledge that some lives are not of equal value. If we stuck rigidly to the letter of the law, which in theory upholds the principle of the sanctity of life and that all lives are equal, then we should be keeping brain dead patients on ventilators indefinitely and prolonging the lives of anencephalic babies.

Certainly in this context, it is hard to see what the value of life is for a patient in a persistent vegetative state, when they have no awareness of themselves, their surroundings or anyone else in the present, and where there is no hope of them ever recovering. But what of those individuals who are conscious, but not rational; who have very limited self-awareness, but who are capable of experiencing pain and pleasure? As Tooley (1986) points out, besides the profoundly mentally impaired people and newborn babies who would be included in this category, many non-human animals would qualify too.

Glover describes different levels of consciousness and asks where, on a sliding scale from merely being aware of sensations to having the capacity for abstract reasoning, do we assess the value of consciousness? In his view being alive has no intrinsic value; life is only valuable if the life is worth living. If to destroy a life that is worth living would be wrong, does it follow that it would not be wrong to destroy a life that is not worth living?

Such views raise significant issues with regard to the growing number of infants who survive the traumas of aggressive treatment and grow up being less than able in those criteria that are deemed necessary to claim an equal right to life. These are the individuals for whom we are concerned. How much are their lives worth in the eyes of society? Are there degrees of worth? How much value is placed on those individuals who do not have the mental capacity to have a great awareness of self or others; who do not see themselves in relation to time or space?

Steven Edwards (1997) argues that society does value intellectually disabled people less, and accords them a lower moral status than those who are intellectually able. He says that the degree of moral status accorded to a class of individuals is apparent, to some degree, in the way we treat and regard those people and the weight of obligations considered due to them. He supports his claim by citing some considerations that he believes show that people with learning disabilities are seen as morally inferior to individuals within the normal range of intelligence.

- The law allows termination of pregnancy on the grounds that the foetus is likely to suffer intellectual disability (e.g. Down's Syndrome). The very fact that it is considered likely the child will be mentally disabled is considered enough grounds for an abortion. The fact that the foetus might otherwise be healthy has no bearing on the decision.
- Until the early 1980s it was considered acceptable practice to withhold nutrition from a baby born with known mental disability, so that it would be left to die. The lawsuit against Dr Leonard Arthur confirmed that doctors considered this 'normal practice' at that time.

• The emerging view of 'personhood' distinguishes a person from a mere human being by certain criteria: awareness of self, awareness of others etc. Here the moral status of the individual is heavily tied into the degree of intellectual awareness they possess.

WHAT IS THE RELEVANCE FOR THE SAVING OF VERY PREMATURE BABIES?

Questions about whether certain lives are more valuable than others, and whether there is such a thing as a life that is not worth living, are very relevant to the dilemmas facing paediatricians in the context of neonatal intensive care. If every child's life is of equal value then each has a right to life-saving or life-sustaining treatment irrespective of their condition or prognosis. However, if Glover's (1977) view is accepted then there will be some babies who will be considered not to have an equal right to treatment. For example, a child born with anencephaly would in normal circumstances be incapable of sustaining independent life for more than a few days, because of the absence of any neurological or natural life support mechanisms.

If all life is intrinsically valuable and everyone deserves equal rights irrespective of their present diagnosis or future prognosis, this infant would be deemed to require equal access to aggressive treatment, which might sustain life indefinitely, but would never restore consciousness or any other human response.

If one took the view that this infant's life was not worth living, because it is not and never could become a conscious being, then morally there would be no reason for trying to treat it or keep it alive. In fact, taking the argument to its limit, it would not be wrong to destroy the life, because it has no intrinsic value. All of these theories are based on the view that what makes life worth living, or what gives life its value, is the possession of certain qualities that together distinguish a *person* from a *human being*.

Wyatt and Spencer (1992) would take the view that all babies' lives have intrinsic value, whether they are disabled or not. Life is a gift from God and its worth does not rely on the potential development of certain characteristics, or its future role within family or society. However badly damaged a baby might be, it still has the right to be treated with the love, respect and dignity that any other person would expect.

According to David Seedhouse (1995), the debate surrounding the sanctity of life principle only serves to prove the irrationality of some judgements made in the neonatal unit. In the end, the decision to withhold or withdraw life support from a severely brain injured infant depends entirely on the beliefs of the Consultant in charge of the case. Seedhouse writes that often the decision to begin treatment, or not, is based more on hunches and feelings than on hard evidence. He cites the example of a very premature neonate, who has had several surgical interventions, is severely damaged and after three months intensive care still cannot breathe without the ventilator. The treatment has probably caused the child much suffering and obviously has not been successful. Seedhouse asserts that this situation has arisen solely because the doctor in charge of the case believes in the sanctity of life doctrine and has complete authority over the treatment. Had a different Consultant been in control at the time, with a different set of values, there could have been a completely different outcome and the child would in all probability have died much sooner.

SANCTITY OF LIFE VERSUS QUALITY OF LIFE ISSUES

As we have seen, supporters of the sanctity of life doctrine hold that it is always wrong to intentionally terminate human life in any circumstances, whatever the quality of that life. For them, all life is equally valuable and inviolable.

We have also noted that this principle is very difficult to maintain in practice, particularly in the field of neonatal intensive care, and even those who subscribe to it feel the need to qualify their arguments in certain circumstances where difficult choices need to be made. Advances in technology and treatments have created challenges for a doctrine that Mason and McCall Smith (1999) describe as rigid and uncompromising in its interpretation. Inevitably, quality of life considerations are taken into account.

Should the sanctity of life principle, based on the deontological principles found within the Hippocratic Oath and in religious doctrines, be replaced by criteria linked to more utilitarian principles based on quality of life considerations?

Singer (1996) argues that the best argument for abandoning the sanctity of life doctrine is its 'sheer absurdity'. He says that if we take the principle seriously, it would mean ignoring all quality of life judgements and that leaves us with the impossible situation of prolonging the lives of anencephalic babies, cortically dead infants and patients in persistent vegetative states.

Singer argues that, today, we have no grounds for saying that all life is of equal value. If someone is unconscious, with no prospect of ever again having any mental, social or physical interaction with other human beings, then that life has little or no value. He also cites the lives of profoundly disabled babies, proposing that harms and benefits should be balanced in decisions about whether they should be allowed to carry on living: will the amount of pain and suffering a multiply disabled child has to bear over a lifetime outweigh the benefits of being conscious and having limited enjoyable experiences with their family and friends? These decisions will have to be faced and everyone involved in the child's care will need to be involved in the decision-making process.

In fact, as we have already established, most decisions made about withdrawing or withholding treatment for babies are based on quality of life criteria. When looking at this from the viewpoint of the sanctity of life doctrine, on which both the law and medicine are supposedly based, it is obvious that ethically they are not mutually tenable. If all human life is valuable and sacrosanct, then it cannot be argued that some lives can be terminated because they are not meaningful.

Milton D Heifetz (1996) states that the quality of life issue has to be faced and makes the very cogent point that in all decision-making processes there is a need to consider the 'whole person', otherwise the doctor may fall into the trap of prescribing aggressive treatment, even if in the long term it will be of no benefit to the child.

> To ignore looking at a newborn as a total human being and instead considering it a body containing a sick organ which is in need of care is a medical anathema.
>
> (Heifetz 1996, p. 147)

Mason and McCall Smith (1999) follow this line and question whether it is good medical practice to keep alive a neonate who is so profoundly disabled that they will never be able to take any meaningful place in society; or one whose life will be full of pain and suffering.

Most agree that in the child's best interests all discussions about his potential or lack of it should be openly discussed with other professionals and parents before crucial decisions are made. Some, like Singer (1996), would suggest that much depends on the wishes of the parents. Taking into account the magnitude of the disabilities, the quality of life for the child will depend largely on their approach and attitude. A desire on their part to nurture and cherish their baby will have a profound effect on its quality of life. Equally, if they feel that the burden of caring for a multiply disabled baby is to much for them or their other children to bear, then it is probable that the child's quality of life would be diminished by being placed in residential care. The future quality of life of any child is affected by parental attitudes towards its care and it is true that some parents cannot commit themselves to rearing an infant who will never be able to fully participate in family life because of crippling mental and physical disabilities. A child who is wanted, even if multiply disabled, will have better quality of life prospects than one who is rejected or abandoned.

Wyatt and Spencer (1992) writing from a distinctively Christian point of view, believe that today the criteria for determining quality of life issues are too much influenced by humanist preoccupations, such as autonomy and the capacity for pleasure. Factors that reduce these functions, such as loss of mobility, loss of sight or dependence on others for everyday needs are seen to represent an unacceptable reduction of the quality of life. Wyatt and Spencer question whether these issues are being over-valued, and suggest that we should be concentrating more on values such as justice, respect and compassion, which would lead to more loving, compassionate and accepting relationships. In this way, disabled individuals would not feel that the rest of society devalued their life.

Wyatt and Spencer make the point that the use of quality of life criteria is fraught with difficulties for any decision maker in a clinical situation. Certainly they believe that parental distress, resource issues and society's attitude to disabled people should never be factors in decisions about whether to withdraw or withhold treatment in the intensive neonatal unit. However, having made the claim that severe disability should not be a factor when considering which course of action to take, paradoxically Wyatt and Spencer do qualify their assertion by adding that there are some situations when it would not be appropriate to continue life support:

> If there is clear and unequivocal evidence of catastrophic global brain injury, intensive care support may be deemed inappropriate.
>
> (Wyatt and Spencer 1992, p. 25)

They add that there should be full agreement of all staff and relatives before the final decision is taken. So, in the end, they are saying that it is appropriate to consider quality of life in extreme cases and that some lives are not worth living.

Robertson (1998) too, feels that any claim that non-treatment is in the child's best interests is questionable. Arguments for allowing the baby to die on the grounds of severe congenital abnormalities, or because the child will suffer a lifetime of physical and emotional stress can be countered, because we cannot know what degree of suffering or distress is too much for another person to endure. Perhaps a child is suffering pain and will need repeated surgery, or other complications may arise, like hydrocephalus, fractures and dislocations. Yet pain may be intermittent and manageable with analgesics. It does not follow that pain alone makes life worthless or not worth living. Neither does the argument that the child will live a life where social interaction is severely limited. Perhaps he/she may suffer parental rejection, may never be able to walk, talk, be independent or make meaningful choices in life. But today many mentally handicapped people can be helped to lead satisfying lives in society. The root of the problem may lie with society's attitude to the care and treatment of the disabled, not with the disabled person themselves. Care and education can help them develop a range of enjoyable and useful activities; so, according to Robertson, arguments that death is preferable to life for some newborn babies cannot be substantiated in most cases. He does not question the sincerity of the parents and doctors who believe that treating such severely disabled infants causes more harm than good. He does question the utilitarian approach that works on the assumption that quality of life (or utility) can be measured and compared with other lives.

There is more at stake here than just the child's quality of life. We are questioning the value of one life against others, making judgements about whose life is more important. In this case the question is whether it is right to save the life of a very severely disabled infant, knowing the devastating impact it will surely have on the quality of life of all the other members of the family.

Heifetz (1996) believes that the concept of 'substituted judgement' can be applied here. Some ethicists prefer the term 'best interests' in the case of a child who has never been autonomous, and whose mental impairment makes it impossible for them to have any wishes to express; but Heifetz argues that it is possible to use a frame of reference from which a substituted judgement can be reached on behalf of the very ill premature baby. He understands that it may be a distressing and harrowing process, particularly for the parents, but it is an essential process, which in the end will always serve the best interests of the baby.

Those who are in the unenviable position of deciding whether a baby's life is worth living or not, have to decide what criteria should be used to make such crucial judgements. They have to determine the criteria that contribute to making a life worth living.

9

Personhood

> There are some groups of children about whose potential we must think more carefully before we allow our moral concern to result in 'heroic' medicine. First there are children who do not have any conscious appreciation of life and will never develop it. They have the physical appearance of human beings, but lack the essential functional qualities of being human, including the capacity for conscious life.
>
> (Campbell, Gillett and Jones 2001, p. 117)

The debate about whether every human being has the right to life, or whether every life is worth living, is closely linked with the question of personhood.

Campbell, Gillett and Jones believe that any baby who fits the above description would have no capacity or potential to appreciate anything in life, including the love and care of others, therefore 'our normal medical concern to treat for recovery can be appropriately suppressed'.

They consider the child is not a person and does not have the capacity for developing those features that are morally relevant to personhood, therefore their life is not worth living and we have no moral obligation to keep them alive.

Others will challenge this view on the principle that all life is of equal value and should be treated with equal respect.

WHAT IS A PERSON?

Some believe that personhood is inherent in every human life from the moment of conception and that at no time is the developing embryo anything else but a real person. Therefore it should be given the same status and right to life as any other human being.

Others claim that being *human* does not necessarily make us a *person*; in order to qualify as a person rather than just a human being it is necessary to possess certain characteristics. For them, personhood is a gradually developing process, for one can hardly say that a bunch of cells in the first few days of human development is a real person; becoming a person as opposed to being merely human is a developmental process and real persons should have a higher status than non-persons. In this case, as Gillon ((1985) points out, the right to life is something owed to people, or persons; therefore if some individuals are not considered persons, then they cannot automatically claim this right. This, of course cuts across the concept of the sanctity of life doctrine.

These opposing viewpoints must inevitably affect the way we value the individual, particularly the growing foetus, the profoundly mentally handicapped person and every newborn baby. If personhood is something which develops gradually over the first few weeks, months or even years after birth, then how do we define it and what characteristics does a human being require to become a real person? Furthermore, is it possible that some individuals will never acquire those characteristics, because of mental retardation, or neurological trauma, or that some will eventually lose those characteristics, as mental faculties deteriorate through age, disease or coma?

One can often hear family and friends describing their developing infant as becoming 'a real little person'. This often happens when the child begins to be aware of himself and others, responding to and initiating responses from those around him. But just as we recognise the developing personality of the growing baby, it is also possible for a family to watch the disintegration of the 'person' they love, in advanced stages of Alzheimer's disease, or in a permanent vegetative state. What then, if anything, distinguishes a person from a mere human being?

Personhood is a gradual development of self-awareness and consciousness

Although 'person' often functions as a synonym for 'human being' there are contexts in which it does not. Hence, although it is trivially true that all human beings are human beings, it is not trivially true that all human beings are persons – some are not.

(Hursthouse 1987, p. 93)

Both Kant and Locke identify certain characteristics that distinguish a person from any other being. These characteristics include the ability to think and make rational decisions, as well as being self aware and conscious of oneself in relation to the past and future, and having the capacity to value one's own life. The rational person, in their view, is responsible for making moral decisions and therefore is owed respect from other rational beings.

Joseph Fletcher, a twentieth century philosopher and humanist, restates the views of these earlier thinkers and said that what makes an individual's life valuable is not their biological structure, but their mental capacities. He listed (1998) fifteen indicators of what he then called 'humanhood', which later became known as 'personhood'. These were criteria for distinguishing a person from a mere human being and included the following:

1. Minimal intelligence
2. Self awareness
3. Self control
4. A sense of time
5. A sense of futurity
6. A sense of past
7. The capability to relate to others
8. Concern for others
9. Communication
10. Control of existence
11. Curiosity
12. Change and changeability
13. Balance of rationality and feeling
14. Idiosyncrasy
15. Neo-cortical function.

Fletcher maintains that his motive, when formulating this list, was to stimulate discussion about how we define what is a person; and certainly many have agreed, disagreed, added to the list or completely rejected his views.

It is obvious that the list he drew up automatically excluded anyone who is not considered a rational being: foetuses, neonates, the mentally disabled and anyone suffering from degenerative mental illness. These individuals are not regarded as persons; therefore they can command no respect or right to life.

Philosopher Michael Tooley (1972) agrees, saying that we have no moral obligation to preserve the life of a developing embryo, foetus or even a newborn baby, because each can be described as a 'thing' not a person.

> There seems little doubt that the newly fertilised ova are not self conscious and equally little doubt that adults are, therefore somewhere along the developmental line, perhaps gradually rather than suddenly, self consciousness must develop.
>
> (Gillon 1985, p. 180)

There are many widely differing suggestions as to when a developing human foetus becomes a person. As we have seen above, for some people there can only be one answer, but for others it is not so simple. The difficulty lies in pinpointing the precise time in gestation when an embryo becomes a person. For some it is when it begins to take on human form; or when it begins to move around spontaneously; or when it reaches viability; or at birth and sometimes even beyond.

In Fletcher's later work he tried to isolate the one essential trait, from all those that he and others named, which could be said to be the one criterion on which all other indicators for personhood were dependent; he called it the *sine qua non* (Fletcher 1988, p. 37): the essential element without which all others were unable to function. From all those traits that he and other others had put forward, four seemed to emerge as frontrunners. They were:

- Neocortical function
- Self-consciousness
- Relational ability
- Happiness.

Michael Tooley considers that self-consciousness is the leader. His view is that when a new baby reaches the age of 10–12 weeks it has begun to lose the reflexes present at birth and has begun to acquire certain attributes of personhood. The Moro reflex and the grasping reflex have been lost and physiological changes in the brain have led to the development of a higher degree of mental functioning. At this point, Tooley believes that although the child has not yet reached the stage of absolute personhood, enough qualities are there to justify him/her some sort of protection.

For Peter Singer (1996) too, the developing embryo is merely a clump of cells; a non-sentient being. Therefore it is of no moral significance for the first few weeks of gestation. For him personhood begins when the growing foetus becomes a sentient being; that is, when it has developed the ability to feel pleasure and pain. Only then does it warrant a moral status and become entitled to protection from anyone who would deliberately inflict pain.

The problem here lies in pinpointing when sentience begins. Is it possible to identify a morally significant dividing line in the developmental process? There are widely differing views about when there is enough neurological development for the foetus to feel pain or sensation. Opinions vary from 6 weeks' gestation to 28 weeks as the point at which a foetus shows the earliest signs of consciousness. If, as some say, the upper limit to complete brain development is around the 28 weeks margin, then this does have significant implications for those babies born at between 23 and 28 weeks' gestation.

Singer's view (1996) is that human life has three groupings:

- **Group 1**: Beings that are alive but not sentient; that is, foetuses under 18 weeks' gestation and certain beings at the very end of life.
- **Group 2**: Beings who are conscious, but not *self-conscious*; that is foetuses over 18 weeks' gestation, young infants and those just conscious, nearing the end of life.
- **Group 3**: These are real 'persons'; they are conscious, rational and self-aware individuals, who see their lives in the context of time (having a past and a future existence).

Fletcher (1998) insists that the basic essential criterion that is the key to personhood must be neocortical function; without the synthesising processes of the cerebral cortex, which enables thought processes and minimal intelligence to function, a being is not a person. The brain stem and mid brain responses, which trigger emotions and regulate autonomic physical functions, are not enough to count when trying to define what is a person.

He illustrates the meaning of his theory, when he describes

(1998, p. 38) how some children with severe learning disabilities and a very low IQ will respond to hugs and touch but are untrainable, although they appear happy in a world of their own; Fletcher likens this state to that of a kitten, which will respond to stroking and show pleasure in the same way.

This illustration does remind me of some of the very young children I taught. A number of the profoundly mentally disabled could be stimulated by the sight or smell of food, or relaxed by a soothing aromatherapy massage. However, apart from these sensory responses they very often showed little or no self-awareness or awareness of others. In fact, one could say that they responded in much the same way as a non-human animal would to touch, taste and smell. Nevertheless, it is possible to see some degree of learning in many of these children, as they get older.

The main teaching programmes with this type of child involve sensory motor stimulation. The growing number of pupils with profound and multiple learning disabilities has triggered much research and training into the development of equipment and techniques to help professionals deliver educational programmes to suit individual needs. Every child has a unique combination of problems, so a multidisciplinary team approach is used to decide the best way to tackle the physical and mental barriers to learning. Although progress is essentially very slow and sometimes painful, staff and parents can sometimes see the fruits of months of patient stimulation with a glimpse of recognition or a response that demonstrates an understanding of what is being experienced. It may just be a flicker of an eyelid or the movement of a limb, indicating a preference when offered a choice of food or activity; however the reaction is registered, if it is rewarded and repeated it can offer some tiny measure of autonomy for that child.

I particularly remember one incident in my classroom with one such pupil. I shall call him Tom.

Tom had been born at 24 weeks' gestation and suffered profound neurological damage, which resulted severe cerebral palsy. Scoliosis of the spine prevented him from sitting up, and he had spasticity of all limbs, so that both gross and fine motor movements of legs, arms, feet and hands were severely restricted. He also suffered from hydrocephalus and had severe visual impairment and learning disabilities. His tiny body was so fragile that he often winced or cried out when handled by carers, however gently we touched him. The one sense that had not been damaged was hearing;

> Tom loved to listen to music, it seemed to soothe him and give him some pleasure.
>
> One morning before school began, I was in my classroom, preparing for the day. Tom always arrived early and this morning I settled him into his special 'work' chair, chatting to him as I fastened all the various straps to keep him comfortable. As usual, he showed little response. When he was ready, I turned on the tape recorder, which was playing a song that the whole school was learning for the Christmas show and which we had been practicing in assembly each afternoon. At one point in the song, the instruments rested and during the silence the children had to tap instruments or clap their hands in a rhythmic response. To my amazement and delight as the tape arrived at the pause, I heard a faint 'tap tapping' on the wooden tray in front of Tom. I turned to look, and he was smiling broadly and his tiny fist was moving in response to the silence in the music. The amount of effort needed for him to achieve that amount of movement was remarkable enough, but the fact that he had responded at the right time in the right place, was more than enough proof that underneath all that damage, was a little person with a great sense of fun.

That was a very moving and satisfying moment and I think it was that incident more than any other that triggered my deep interest in the concept of personhood.

Human persons and non-human persons

Although Singer (1996) identifies three morally significant groups, in his view it is not possible to distinguish between our own human species and any other. He maintains that all three categories can be found in a number of species, not only in human beings. Jane Goodall's (1986) work observing the habits and lifestyle of chimpanzees and Francine Patterson and Wendy Gordon's (1994) description of the characteristics of Koko the gorilla lend support to Singer's theories. These non-human animals display characteristics showing them to be intelligent, thinking individuals who understand language and show the same sort of emotions as a human person.

Singer illustrates his premise with an account taken from some observations made by Jane Goodall:

> A group of people were observed living their everyday lives in a new type of institution, set in a large two-acre site, in the Netherlands. These people were unable to speak and although physically able, they were operating well below the normal human mental capacity. Nevertheless their communication skills were quite considerable, and they managed to make themselves

understood to each other through gestures and sounds.

Despite these problems they soon devised their own ways of dealing with problems: a leader emerged, who arbitrated on disagreements. He had privileges but also obligations to the group. They developed a certain ethical code of behaviour: helping each other with problems and punishing wrongdoing.

They were not a monogamous group, so it was not always possible to know who had fathered which children. They had little to do with the nurturing of the offspring, but the mothers were competent and caring and the mother/child relationships were very close.

One of the older mothers appeared to take on the matriarchal role, showing the younger ones techniques for controlling unruly behaviour in the young.

They were given maximum freedom to explore the grounds, which were surrounded by a high wall. At one point some of the group formed an escape party, and used branches from trees propped up against the wall to try and escape.

The results of this study showed that despite their limited mental capacity, they were able to devise strategies for living and problem solving, including devious tactics to avoid trouble or enlist sympathy from other members of the group.

The point of this discourse is that Singer has referred to them throughout as 'people'; collectively they have displayed characteristics of self-awareness and rational thought, which he asserts are essential to personhood. However, as you may have guessed, these 'people' are in fact not members of the human species who suffer from severe learning disabilities; they are actually members of the species *Pan troglodytes*, a group of chimpanzees, living in Arnhem Zoo. Jane Goodall's observations showed that they were able to plan future behaviour, evidence that they were both self-conscious and capable of rational thought.

The point Singer makes is that if some members of another species can show the same characteristics as some human beings, why is it that we see their lives as being somehow less morally significant? The root of the problem lies in the fact we tend to use the expressions 'persons' and 'human beings' interchangeably. For those who share Singer's analysis, this is a fundamental mistake; all life, whether human or not, has the same moral significance and should be treated with equal respect. Singer's philosophy is that there are other species, apart from humans, who will be sentient beings; others may display characteristics of personhood which may not be present in some members of the human race. Singer's very controversial view is that we have made comparisons between severely mentally disabled individuals and some non-human animals taboo, to preserve the boundaries surrounding the sanctity of life doctrine, which gives human beings a totally different moral status than any other species, whether or not they display any characteristics of personhood.

According to this view of personhood, although some individuals are humans, they do not necessarily qualify as persons too. Some are sentient but not self-conscious, and that includes the very premature neonate, with whom we are concerned. If this is the case, what are the implications for our treatment and care of humans who would not qualify as persons?

What, for example is our attitude towards members of another species when they are known to be in pain and suffering from an incurable disease?

Our own faithful and much loved family pet, Fergus, a 12-year-old golden retriever, was a conscious being; whether he was self-conscious is questionable. At the end of his life he was in a great deal of distress, suffering from an enlarged heart and failing kidneys. We kept hoping that he would die peacefully, but he kept living for weeks, getting more and more bloated and struggling to breathe. In the end the vet's words were: 'He has been a faithful friend to you: now it is your turn to be the best friend to him. It is time to let him go.' The decision was awful, but we consented to have him put down humanely, to alleviate any further misery at the end of his life.

Looking at the concept of personhood from this perspective, why is it morally permissible to actively alleviate the suffering of one species of sentient beings, by giving them a painless injection to hasten death in a futile situation, but unethical to treat a member of another species in the same way? Why is it that our moral thinking distinguishes how we treat human beings who could be classed as members of Singer's first two groupings, from any other species categorised in the same way?

Why is it considered morally wrong to give a simple injection to a human person for whom there is no hope of recovery, and who is in great distress, when we are expected to act in exactly the opposite way for a non-human? Both Tooley (1972) and Singer (1996) maintain that it is very difficult to defend such inconsistencies in reasoning.

However, there is another problem. Again I remember from my own teaching experience cases of children who were much more puzzling when it came to defining personhood. In particular, I recall one seven-year-old girl; a pretty child, dark eyed and long limbed. Physically she was completely normal. Her birth had been uneventful at full term, with no complications and no abnormalities detected. She was discharged from hospital in the normal way and no problems were reported from home during the first few months of life. Everything seemed fine, until she began to fall behind on some of the cognitive milestone tests. Hearing and sight tests were carried out, but again everything seemed normal. Physically she sat up and learned to walk within average limits, but she began falling behind more and more in speech and cognitive ability. In fact her speech was non-existent; she never made babbling sounds or uttered baby talk and showed little interest in reaching or grabbing for toys or food. As she developed into a toddler, she never learned to use her potty and became more and more hyperactive. Her mother, in particular, found it very hard to admit that there was anything wrong, because there were no physical signs of abnormality. Eventually, however, she was given a statement of educational needs and was sent to a school for children with severe learning disabilities.

She appeared to be completely unaware of herself and showed no recognition of others, not even her family members. She did not speak or respond to her name, never smiled or cried and showed no interest in toys or books. Even music, which is often a wonderful stimulus for children with special needs, had no effect on her at all. She showed no motivation to feed herself, even though there was absolutely no physical reason why she could not do this. She would eat food that was offered from a spoon, but showed neither enjoyment nor dislike of the taste. She remained doubly incontinent. Every few minutes she would get up and run around the room, or out of the door if it was open. Taking her out into the community was a nightmare, for she had no sense of danger and would take off if her carer loosed her hand for a second. Not once, in the five years I taught her, did she respond to anything that we tried; eye contact was fleeting and it almost appeared that her mind was a complete blank, with no awareness of self or others, and no concept of time or space. In comparison to some of the most severe cases of cerebral palsy, even those children who had suffered massive brain injury, I found her the most frustrating to teach; although her physical development continued quite normally, mentally she appeared to be entirely without any vestige of personhood as described by Fletcher (1998), Tooley (1972) or Singer (1996). I am fairly sure that she did not have the capacity to value her own life. Her life appeared to be biological but not biographical; she was certainly conscious, but not self-conscious. Yet I am sure that no one would seriously question her entitlement to the same protection and right to life as any other individual.

A POTENTIAL PERSON

Whatever we now are was present in potential form in the embryos from which we developed.

(Campbell, Gillett and Jones 2001, p. 102)

This view of the development of personhood sees the foetus as a being with the potential to become a fully aware conscious person. It has the capacity for personhood, and therefore has a claim to respect and life. No arbitrary lines are drawn before or after certain stages of development; in every stage, however rudimentary, the human foetus is progressing to personhood. So, since there is a continuous line of human development from fertilisation through to birth, childhood and the fully-grown adult, at what point can we say that it is morally permissible to destroy that person?

Some argue that as each developmental stage is reached the rights of the foetus to respect and life get stronger so that, in the final stages of pregnancy, it has the same status as an actual person. Gillon (1985) believes that this is the case and that because the development of the foetus towards a rational, self-conscious being is a gradual process, there are plausible reasons why society should also give a 'gradually increasing moral protection to the developing embryo, foetus and newly born infant' (p. 181). The wrongness of destroying either a human foetus or very young baby lies in the fact that they are being deprived of the chance to develop all their human potential. But what of the babies whom we feel may not be capable of reaching that full potential; the babies who are born with profound disabilities and the very premature infant damaged by aggressive measures to save its life?

Walters (1988) further extends the idea of a potential person and puts forward the idea of 'approximate personhood'. In order to aid decision making in difficult situations, he proposes that at birth all these marginal cases should be assessed for their potential to develop the capabilities of personhood by a paediatrician. If their abnormalities approximate to a reasonable chance of attaining this, then he suggests that the child should receive appropriate treatment. In effect this would mean that any child with minor disabilities would always be treated, but parents would be consulted as to the best way forward for those with more severe problems. Of course, one could begin to ask what capabilities Walters has in mind in order to qualify for 'approximate personhood', and it would probably be very difficult to find two paediatricians whose views were precisely in line for marginal cases.

Celia Wells (1989) points to the difficulties with the potentiality theory: although it may seem attractive and plausible at first, one is forced to ask the same questions as before. How far back can we go with potentiality? The difficulties still exist as to when the developing embryo takes on the status of a potential person: is it from the moment of conception, or somewhere along the line, through the other stages mentioned earlier?

All humans are persons from the moment of fertilisation to the day they die

> Science and philosophy concur in the conclusion: every human individual must be regarded as a person.
>
> (Finnis 1999, p. 15)

John Finnis (1999) argues that there is no difference between a human being and a person. Human beings are persons by the very nature of their being born to human parents. From the very beginning, the biological capacity to support all kinds of human operations is carried in the genetic code of all fertilised human ova. These potential activities are distinctive to the human species and include all those criteria that can be included to describe a human person.

The fact that a human foetus takes on the physical characteristics of a human being very early in gestation is enough to confirm its right to personhood. As early as the tenth week of pregnancy the foetus has developed arms, legs, fingers and toes; internal organs are developing and there is evidence of primitive brain function.

Therefore Finnis proposes that at the very onset of life a foetus is not just a potential person, but in fact is a 'human person with potential'. So an individual has a truly human nature from the moment of fertilisation. How is it possible to differentiate between a full term child just before and just after birth; and is it even possible to say that the full term baby is not the same individual person as it was three months, six months, or even nine months earlier in the womb? From the earliest stage of development the embryo should be entitled to the same treatment as a fully-grown person. Therefore, if we accept that a foetus is a person, it then follows that it is permitted the full legal rights, privileges and respect due to any other human person, whether they be competent or incompetent.

Those who appose abortion accept this view, believing that the right of a foetus to life will always have precedent over a woman's right to choose, because killing a foetus is in fact killing a person and therefore is morally unjustifiable. Abortion, whether for social or personal reasons, is ethically unacceptable.

There is also the view that the idea of non-personhood, at any age, refutes the right of disabled people to be seen as equal citizens in a just and caring society. Wyatt and Spencer (1992) subscribe to this view and are firm in their Christian view that all humans are made in the image of God, which makes their life intrinsically valuable irrespective of any physical or mental abnormality.

PREMATURE BABIES: PERSONHOOD AND RIGHT TO LIFE

According to Singer (1996), Tooley (1972) and others, personhood is the key to deciding whether an individual has the right to life. In their view, being a person involves the capacity to be aware of oneself and others and having a concept of our existence in time, so that we see ourselves in the context of past and future experiences; we can have a will and desire to look forward to what the future holds for us. If such an person should expressly wish to live, then it would be wrong and a violation of their human rights to end the life of that person, for they would have been denied the opportunity to fulfil any future plans or ambitions that they may have been looking forward to. Age is not an issue here, for even the very old may still have a strong desire to live to see some future event which is of great importance to them.

An individual who does not possess these faculties is not a person: they are not aware of themselves or of others and are incapable of possessing any views or desires about whether their lives should continue or not. They cannot look back on any events in their life or forward to any future possibilities. If this is the case, the argument continues, it would be less serious to end such a life. If the human being is incapable of knowing that its life has value and meaning and has no capacity for looking back on their life or anticipating the future, they cannot have a will to live. Therefore, morally, their life is no more valuable or worthy of protection than that of a foetus.

The very premature neonate can be described as a biological but not a biographical human being. Indeed, it could be said that no newborn infant could be seen as a person if valued against these criteria. If this is the case the argument against infanticide becomes irrelevant, for the arguments used to support abortion can easily be extrapolated to justify the non-treatment or even killing of any newborn, whether disabled or not. As we have seen in the arguments above, if they are not persons, they have no right to life. It is for this reason that many people defend the sanctity of life principle, in the belief that by abandoning it we are moving closer to the 'slippery slope' where selective treatment might be used on babies for trivial reasons, like being the wrong sex or having the wrong colour eyes.

It is true that in some cultures, even today, the value and right to life of babies, particularly those born prematurely or with disabilities, is not seen as equal to that of older children or adults. Singer (1996) cites the Japanese traditional practice of 'mabiki' or 'thinning' of infants. When a child was born, particularly one with disabilities, there was no underlying assumption that it should continue to live. The midwife would ask whether the infant was 'to be left' or 'to be returned' (sent back to the place from whence it came; wherever they believed that to be). Invariably, the child with disabilities was 'returned'. Tooley (1972) also makes the point that in our society too, those who are considering the future of a baby who has not yet reached the stage of self-awareness, have fewer problems making decisions about treatment than when considering older or more able children. It is certainly true that examples of this attitude can be found in law. The parents of the baby with Down's Syndrome in the case of Dr Leonard Arthur were quite adamant in their rejection of the child whom they regarded as less than perfect. They were insistent that the child should not live and the paediatrician was quite happy to go along with their decision. One wonders, however, what the parents' feelings would have been if the child had been allowed to live for a few weeks and they had given themselves time to get to know him. Would they have still been able to make the same decision? How can doctors justify the actions that lead to the death of such a baby, when they would almost certainly reject such a course of treatment for an older Down's Syndrome patient?

These attitudes towards the newborn certainly give the impression that their lives are not considered in the same light as those who have grown into 'little people'.

Singer (1996) raises an interesting point that has some relevance to that question. He refers to the ancient Greek tradition of allowing a period of time to elapse between the birth of a baby and a ceremony that bestowed the status of personhood onto the child and marked the parents' formal decision to accept the child. He suggests that our society might well adopt such a system whereby a period of possibly 28 days after birth is allowed, in which the child's future may be assessed. Only after that period is the child recognised as having the same right to life as anyone else. Singer admits that there are problems when one begins to lay down boundaries and markers for decisions about when a human being becomes a person, and has a right to life. Nevertheless the only marker we have at present is the moment of birth; and because the limits of viability of the foetus are being constantly challenged, decision making at the very beginning of life is becoming more and more difficult. Parents and doctors are facing enormous dilemmas about whether to withhold or withdraw treatment. Perhaps a period of consideration immediately after birth would give everyone the chance to make crucial decisions about whether or not to continue to support that life, before any official status or right to existence is conferred on it.

Many people would argue that tiny infants, whether or not they are handicapped, whether or not they are real persons, belong to the human species, and most have the potential to become persons, means that they should have the same right to protection as anyone else. Robertson (1998) feels that the human species is sufficiently different from other sentient species to automatically give its members greater rights at birth. Wells (1989) also dispels ideas against distinguishing between species when she makes the analogy between a human embryo that has the potential to develop into a fully-grown person and an acorn that has the potential to become a mighty oak tree. One cannot say that the acorn is the same thing as an oak tree but it has more in common with an oak tree than does a privet hedge; in the same way a human foetus may not be regarded as a person, but it has more in common with a human person than, for example, a caterpillar.

However, like Singer, Robertson does qualify this by saying that there might be persuasive arguments according them less protection than a fully fledged person; many people actually do regard disabled newborns in a different light than older children. Just as the destruction of an acorn is in no way like the destruction of an oak tree, for many people the destruction of a non-person is seen as less of a problem than the destruction of a person.

The law tells us that technically a foetus born before 24 weeks' gestation is not viable, therefore we have no legal obligation to save it. We know, however, that up-to-the-minute expertise is making it possible to save foetuses before that date. It is here that the law, ethics and technology have reached an impasse: it is justifiable ethically and legally to abort foetuses which are abnormal, for example those diagnosed with Down's Syndrome, but not legally or morally permissible to humanely kill a premature newborn or full term Down's Syndrome baby.

Even though some people may not regard neonates, whether premature or full term, as persons, this does not mean that they are not entitled to some protection. As Gillon (1985) points out, families and society in general place great value on the life of a new baby; much more than they put on foetuses and embryos. The event of giving birth does mark a change in our feelings and attitude. The status of the foetus is altered in our perception at that point and even those who find abortion acceptable would be horrified at the idea of terminating the life of a newborn. As Wells (1989) says, few people find indiscriminate killing of any living human being, including foetuses or newborn babies, acceptable. Most people would find it abhorrent and morally wrong to deliberately kill a healthy infant.

The question is, do we place equal value on the life of a very premature baby with a poor prognosis? From Wyatt and

Spencer's (1992) point of view there is no doubt that even a very damaged baby is fully human and deserves protection. Campbell, Gillett and Jones (2001) also state that as humans we have a deep commitment to the care and protection of our own species. The human infant appeals to our moral feeling of responsibility for the nurture of that child. Robertson (1998) does not believe that withholding treatment for seriously disabled infants can be justified; he argues that to hold this view assumes that newly born infants can be classified into two different kinds of offspring: those which are persons and those which are not. If one begins to qualify criteria which distinguish a person from a non-person, then there is a danger of opening the door to abuse and suffering for those who are considered less than human. Robertson reminds us that slavery, witch-hunts and wars have been justified on the grounds that the victims were less than human. Therefore, we should presume personhood for all newborn infants, irrespective of whether they are damaged or not, because trying to define specific characteristics or criteria that might exclude some of them may lead to malpractice and abuse. Robertson points out how difficult it can be to predict which babies will develop self-awareness: only those infants with anencephaly or massive brain trauma will never develop any sense of self.

However, Campbell, Gillett and Jones (2001) caution that there are some groups of children who may have the physical appearance of human beings, but who lack the potential to develop the functional qualities that they need to become fully human. They will never have the capacity to appreciate whether things matter to them or not. In these cases they maintain that we as a society are released from any obligation to keep such children alive.

So to summarise, some say that if a newborn infant does not have the potentiality for full personhood then ethically there are no arguments for treating the child. Others go further by arguing that in these circumstances it is in the child's best interests not to be allowed to develop into a severely disabled human being. Nevertheless, even though they may not be entitled to full protection or a right to life, like any sentient being they do have the right to be protected from unnecessary pain and suffering.

Others will argue that any newborn baby is a potential person and has the same right to life as any other person. The potentiality argument can work both ways: either it is used to support the arguments for protecting the right to life of the very premature baby on the grounds that the child is a potential member of the human race, or it is used to argue the case that killing a foetus or a neonate is not the same thing as killing a human person.

Does an extremely premature neonate have the same moral status as a foetus, or should it be protected like any full term baby? If it is permissible to terminate the life of a foetus of 22 weeks' gestation, why is it wrong to actively kill an extremely premature baby of the same gestational age, if both are judged to be non-persons?

Recently I was driving behind a car that a stickers in the back window, which read 'Tiny person on board'. It made me think. The notice did not say 'Baby on board' as some do; it did not announce 'tiny human being on board'. The use of the phrase 'tiny person' made me wonder whether as a society we are becoming more accepting of the idea that very young infants are actually persons in their own right, even those who are extremely premature; and whether this has something to do with the very fact that we are now able to see them surviving against all odds as a result of increasingly advanced technology and knowledge, and quickly becoming part of a loving family.

Years ago, when a 23 or 24-week-old foetus was 'miscarried' no one outside the maternity staff saw it, sometimes not even the mother. It was usually taken away and disposed of without any kind of ceremony. Nowadays, if a premature infant, however early, dies during birth, parents are encouraged to hold and cuddle it and say goodbye in their own way. The baby's death is treated in just the same way as if it had been any other older child in the family. Sometimes photographs are taken and the child may be named; parents are asked whether they would like a proper funeral. I know of one funeral director who specialises in these services and charges little or nothing for the facility.

> I noticed something about the reaction to the Chancellor's (Gordon Brown's) baby, which wouldn't have been true 20 years ago. The public accepted that Jennifer Brown was a person who died. Whereas my mother's generation would have thought of a premature child as not quite a person.
>
> (Summers 2002, p. 41)

This observation made by Marie Hillett, Chairperson of the charity BLISS, following the much publicised death of Gordon and Sarah Brown's very premature baby, seems to confirm the view that public perception about the personhood of very premature infants has undergone a subtle change over recent years. Perhaps this is because neonatology has improved their chances of surviving at earlier and earlier gestational age. People can now identify with them, just like any other newly born baby, seeing their potentiality as human persons.

This was brought home to me very movingly during my work as a teacher of children with severe learning disabilities. One of the children in my group, David, was very profoundly disabled and a member of a loving and lively family with two other children, both absolutely normal. When the mother became pregnant with her fourth child, she was routinely scanned at 16 weeks. Sadly, this revealed that the foetus she was carrying had a chromosomal abnormality that was unrelated to David's disabilities. This cruel fluke of nature was a terrible blow to the parents, who were devastated by the news. Doctors were certain that the two conditions were totally unconnected and that it was purely coincidental that this should have happened to them again. The parents decided to leave things for a month in the hope of finding out the extent of the harm to the foetus; but unfortunately at 20 weeks another ultrasound scan revealed severe damage and a termination was recommended. Both parents went through agonies of self-blame and anguish about what to do next, but in the end decided that they really could not cope with another severely handicapped child.

A termination was performed at 21 weeks and the tiny neonate was baptised, but died within minutes of birth. I was invited to the funeral service in a local church, where a photograph of the baby was displayed on the tiny coffin. It was a most moving occasion and all the family, including grandparents, were there to mourn their loss. There was no doubt at all in the eyes of the family and church that even though his life had been deliberately terminated, they were burying a little person; a much loved member of their family.

10

The slippery slope argument

> The slippery slope may refer either to a prediction about empirical consequences if some moral change occurs, or to a linkage in reasoning if certain premises are accepted.
>
> (Pence 1995, p. 30)

Pence (1995) describes the slippery slope as a metaphor that has become a very powerful image in ethics and politics. He portrays an issue or situation as resting on the edge of a steep slope and moral principles as chocks or wedges that prevent it from sliding down. If we take away one or more chocks, this will set off a downward slide that may be imperceptible at first, but then it will gain momentum. The force could dislodge more chocks until the slide becomes unstoppable and ends in disaster at the bottom of the slope, which represents moral chaos or ruin. Other metaphors that have been used to describe the same type of events are 'a foot in the door', or 'the thin end of the wedge'.

Recent debates surrounding so-called 'designer babies' clearly illustrate the way that the slippery slope image is used: in February 2002 the Human Fertilisation and Embryology Authority gave a landmark ruling that it was ethically permissible for a couple from Leeds to select an embryo to implant in the mother, so that tissue from the new baby would match that of their first child, who was suffering from the rare blood disease beta thalassaemia major. The disease is incurable and the child's only chance of survival was through a bone marrow transplant, but a matching donor could not be found. The parents decided that in order to save the life of their child, they would try to conceive another child who would be a genetic match. Blood taken from the umbilical cord could then be transplanted into the sick child and the complications associated with rejection of foreign tissue would be eliminated.

The Authority took 18 months to reach their controversial decision, and insisted that it was a 'one off' ruling, which would not set a precedent. They laid down strict criteria by which other cases may be considered in the future, emphasising that this action was only ethically acceptable in certain circumstances. However, those who opposed the ruling warned that this was the slippery slope and the decision would open the floodgates to all sorts of other practices. They cautioned that in the future other parents would surely follow suit and 'designer' babies could be created to supply spare parts for many other medical conditions. Babies have the right to be valued for themselves alone, not just for their worth as a means of saving someone else's life.

Others, in favour of the ruling, believed we should use advancing knowledge, expertise and technology for the good of society. If the means to save lives are available, it would be wrong not to use them, particularly where a young child is concerned.

So the debate is polarised. Should we take the risk of removing some of the ethical 'chocks' which preserve the status quo, so that children's lives may be saved, but in doing so, weaken other moral safeguards which could fall, opening the door to malpractice and misuse of power?

HOW DOES THE ARGUMENT APPLY TO SAVING VERY PREMATURE BABIES?

The slippery slope debate which surrounds the issues of euthanasia and withdrawing or withholding treatment, is particularly relevant in the case of the plight of the very ill premature baby. It can be viewed from two perspectives.

View 1

> If you accept quality of life as the standard, then first you withdraw the respirators, then the food and then you actively kill people, it's a straight line from one place to the others.
>
> (Pence 1995, p. 83)

Pence is quoting a spokesman for the Right to Life organisation. Supporters of this premise argue that if legislation were to be introduced permitting mercy killing on the grounds of 'quality of life considerations' (whether for an adult or a newborn baby), there could, over time, be a general decline in respect for human life. There could be subtle changes in the general attitude towards the chronically sick and elderly, or the physically and mentally impaired adult or child. What may start off as a humane act could finish up as a vehicle for killing those who may become a burden on society for social or economic reasons. Some have warned of these dangers in the context of Hitler's treatment of the Jews and any other human who did not fit his particular view about the type of people who should make up the 'master race'. They advise caution when considering legislation to allow the practice of euthanasia. In the case of impaired neonates, they fear that parents may start to choose, on the one hand, to withhold treatment for far less serious conditions, or on the other hand, to demand resuscitation of younger and younger foetuses.

David Lamb (1988) uses the 'thin end of the wedge' metaphor. He cautions those who propose new boundaries in good faith to beware of those whose motives are not so pure, and warns against dismissing the sanctity of life doctrine too lightly. There are, he feels, problems with Kohl's (1974) view that people are capable of compartmentalising and rationalising. While the idea may appear fine in theory, problems could arise in practice, like the need to spell out what exactly is meant by 'categories' or 'classes'. Woolly edges may lead to exploitation or the pushing out of boundaries by those with dubious motives of their own. He describes difficulties in deciding how boundaries between categories would be drawn up and how a precise definition of what counts as a 'merciful death' would be achieved. He also sees huge problems involved in deciding what qualities would be needed in order for an individual to have a 'life worth living', for there are bound to be wide discrepancies of opinion on these matters.

View 2

The merciful killing of patients who want to die, does not necessarily lead to the killing of the unwanted or the extermination of the human species.

(Kohl 1974, p. 20)

Kohl (1974), a proponent of voluntary euthanasia and abortion, counters that although we may see possible adverse consequences following from the original argument, those consequences may not actually happen. If euthanasia were legalised or became morally acceptable it does not follow that all sorts of bad consequences or abuse would arise. Kohl contends that rational human beings are able to compartmentalise and limit their generalisations, citing the example of the 'same kind' or 'same class': if one kills an insect, believing it to be a permissible act, it does not follow that one goes on from there to assume that it is permissible to kill all living things. It is far more likely that the individual will limit the generalisation to that particular insect or group of creatures.

Harris (1985) disputes the appropriateness of the Nazi analogy, making the point that the motives of a doctor who is considering whether to withdraw or withhold treatment from a very ill baby, are entirely different from those involved in Hitler's extermination programme during the holocaust. It is precisely because parents and doctors care deeply about the welfare of the child that they may decide that further treatment will only add to its suffering. The treatment that Jews and mentally subnormal people received in concentration camps could never be seen as in their own best interests; therefore the two situations cannot be compared.

Singer (1996), too, rejects the slippery slope argument and focuses attention on the problems for those making difficult decisions in the field of neonatal special care. He questions the argument that by abandoning the sanctity of life doctrine we risk bad consequences, saying that we may actually be submitting innocent babies to suffer more harm by needlessly keeping them alive in futile situations.

Neil Campbell (1999) goes as far as to say that slippery slope arguments against euthanasia, in the case of severely disabled and very sick babies who are aware of pain, are unjust arguments. His view is that the symptoms resulting from the withdrawal of some aggressive treatments are painful, and until the child loses consciousness it may be suffering considerable distress. To alleviate suffering, large amounts of analgesics, probably morphine, are often prescribed. These will almost certainly result in the child ceasing to breathe, but Campbell firmly believes that in the child's best interest, this is the only ethical course of action to take. Though Campbell acknowledges that the line between active euthanasia and relieving pain is very fine, he feels that in circumstances such as this, doctors should have the courage to do what is best for their patient.

Some people argue that to allow parents to make the final choices about withdrawing or withholding treatment for their very ill baby would be to open the door to all sorts of abuse of that right. Parents may choose to withhold treatment from babies who have potential to live a good life, or may demand resuscitation of younger and younger foetuses. Davies (2001) rejects this argument, pointing out that for many parents and babies, life or death decisions do not arise because there is no question about what is in the child's best interest. They only arise when the most suitable treatment and the best option are far from clear. When a baby has a significant chance of a healthy survival then there will be no doubt as to which course of action to take: medical treatment and/or intervention would unquestionably be in the child's best interest. Likewise, if the outlook and prognosis is so poor that the chance of survival without profound disabilities is uncertain, it is likely that further intervention would not be in the child's best interest.

In both of these extremes, the options are clear and decisions are straightforward. However, when there are no easy answers and options are not straightforward, parents should be allowed to make the final complex and unselfish judgement.

SO WHERE DO WE GO FROM HERE?

Slippery slope arguments compel us to examine whether unacceptable harms may ensue from good intentions and sometimes exciting initial decisions. They also remind us that once a practice is made legal or condoned, a line has been drawn which can never again be redrawn.

Harris (1985) takes the view that slopes are only slippery if they catch us unawares and we have ventured onto them without proper equipment. Nevertheless, he also warns that we are only able to identify slippery slopes when we are already on them. Harris makes the point that it would be irrational and immoral to ignore new and potentially beneficial developments in technology and medicine, because we are afraid that in the future, someone who is less scrupulous may try to misuse the knowledge. We should have the courage to follow the route we believe to be right, and to speak out against any future malpractice.

PART 4

Should the baby live?

Part 4 looks at the unique dilemmas in neonatal intensive care, and at the ongoing debate over responsibility for decision-making.

PART CONTENTS

11

Withholding and withdrawing treatment

Decisions about whether to begin or withhold treatment immediately after birth are, by necessity, made very quickly and under extreme pressure. The problem for the doctors is that once a course of treatment is started, it is potentially difficult to abandon it, for expectations are raised and pressure to continue, even in futile circumstances, is high. On the other hand, if aggressive measures are not tried in the first place, some may claim that the baby is not being given a fair and proper chance; it also buys time for a more thorough diagnosis and assessment to be made.

This section considers the dilemmas that confront doctors, nurses and parents immediately following the birth of a very premature baby, and outlines certain doctrines that have evolved and act as an ethical framework to help practitioners make crucial clinical decisions.

Hamish is a premature infant weighing only 536g. He lies in an incubator wired up to a battery of machines hissing and whirring, alarms occasionally disturbing the rhythmic background sounds. His skin is grey, stretched tightly over his bony frame. His abdomen is grossly distended and dark brown exudates seeps into a bag lying on the mattress. Eight adults, all except one wearing light blue trouser suits, stand looking at his laboured breathing, their expressions betraying their concern. The twelve days since his precipitate delivery have been full of invasive procedures and grave prognoses. Scans reveal that his brain is severely damaged. Lungs and intestine show serious problems.

Hamish's parents sit silently on low chairs hedged into a corner, to one side of the circle of uniformed doctors and nurses. They do not look into the eyes of the consultant neonatologist when he addresses them. Everyone is thinking the same question: should we continue to treat him? Is it in Hamish's own best interests? And all over the country the question is repeated, though the babies are all unique, and the circumstances all slightly different.

(McHaffie and Fowlie 1996, p. 1)

The plight of Hamish illustrates the problems involved when a very premature baby with a very low birth weight is saved in the first few minutes after birth, then subsequently develops multiple and profound disabilities. It highlights the dilemma facing doctors and parents about whether to begin or withhold treatment at the very outset.

DILEMMAS IN NEONATAL SPECIAL CARE

Withholding treatment

Selective treatment of very premature babies

According to Mason and McCall Smith (1999) the issue of selective treatment of the neonate is closely tied to the subject of abortion. It is legally permissible to terminate the life of a foetus that has been diagnosed in utero as imperfect, right up to the end of pregnancy. What, then, is to become of those undiagnosed in pregnancy but born prematurely and with some sort of disorder? If it is officially acceptable to abort an imperfect foetus at any stage of pregnancy, why are doctors not permitted to actively end the life of a very premature baby with multiple disabilities?

Many practitioners are seriously questioning whether all preterm babies should be treated in intensive care or whether the use of technology is too indiscriminate. The very fact of their extreme prematurity means that the condition of these babies will be critical immediately following birth and they will need mechanical ventilation, extra oxygen and many other life-saving treatments. Even then death may be inevitable, and for those who survive there is a high risk of severe neurological damage. Some doctors believe that the long term risks are too great, for even those children who survive without physical disabilities have other problems; they are more likely to need special education, for they have lower IQ scores than other children, and exhibit psychiatric disorders, attention deficit, hyperactivity, depression, anxiety and antisocial behaviour. Some doctors believe that in the child's best interest, it is better to withhold treatment at the very outset, before the situation becomes more complicated.

Resource issues are also a concern in discussions about selective treatment. The section in this book on justice and resources illustrates how paediatricians are painfully aware of the implications of saving infants with low gestational age and very low birth weight. Often, these babies will block beds, so that larger babies born afterwards, who may have a greater chance of living without disability, are harmed or die because of lack of resources. For that reason alone, many doctors will justify the selection of some premature babies for treatment, while leaving others to simply survive for as long as they can.

This practice may appear unethical: decisions about non-treatment mean that doctors are, in essence, responsible for the death of some infants. However, harsh realities have to be faced in a situation of limited resources and staff shortages and it is hard to see how else they could act. The judgement about which babies to treat should not make the decision maker responsible for the death of those who are left, even though it may have been foreseen. Doctors cannot be held responsible for shortage of cots or of trained staff.

Kuhse and Singer (1985) surveyed 200 obstetricians and paediatricians in Victoria, Australia. The vast majority (198) agreed it was appropriate, in some circumstances, *not* to use all available means to keep a very ill neonate alive; but only 31% of obstetricians and 40% of paediatricians thought active euthanasia was justified. So, 99% would allow a baby to die, but over 60% could not actively kill the child.

Sometimes parental consent is not sought to begin treatment, because of the necessary speed and the context in which decisions have to be made. The birth has often been so traumatic and precipitous that parents are often ill prepared to face such decisions, for which they have had no prior warning. Therefore they are heavily reliant on the advice and experience of medical staff regarding which course of action might be appropriate for their baby. They do not have the knowledge or experience to disagree with whatever treatment is chosen, so are obliged to place all their trust in the doctor's decision.

However, parents' views are usually considered if there is a need to decide whether to withdraw the treatment. By that point, there has been some time for doctors to explain the full picture about the child's condition and parents are in a better position to make their feelings known.

Practices vary from hospital to hospital and can depend on the particular viewpoint of the paediatrician in charge. Where intensive care is used more selectively, the Consultant makes a judgement about whether he feels aggressive treatment would be beneficial, before it is started. In some cases, the child receives nursing care only, with the parents handling, cuddling and having whatever contact they wish. The baby is allowed to die without the interference of any medical or surgical procedures.

Ideally, decisions about the treatment of a premature baby would be made before delivery; doctor and parents could discuss the various options open to them depending on the condition and gestation of the infant at birth. However, if the premature birth is not expected and delivery is fairly rapid, the decision about whether to begin treatment is often made by whichever junior doctor happens to be on call at that time. Clear guidelines need to be laid down so that all staff understand when *not* to attempt resuscitation; withdrawing treatment can be a complicated and distressing option.

Criteria used in selective treatment

The primary criteria used for selective treatment are birth weight and gestational age. Babies who weigh less than 500 grams are rarely treated by aggressive means. Gestational age may also be considered if it is known for certain, and if the treatment can be planned before the birth.

Wyatt and Spencer (1992) make the point that because gestational age is of such importance in assessing the prognosis for these infants, all borderline cases should be examined to establish the correct gestational age immediately after birth. For babies born at less than 23 weeks' gestational age (or any slightly above 23 weeks who are in poor condition) the outlook is hopeless and they have no chance of long-term survival so resuscitation is withheld. However Wyatt and Spencer do add the proviso that if there is any doubt at all that the child might respond, appropriate measures should be taken.

Different criteria emerge when the problem of scarce resources is a reality. In this case it could be appropriate to withhold intensive treatment of infants born at less than 26 weeks' gestation or of less than 750 grams birth weight in the expectation that they would die shortly after birth anyway. Wyatt and Spencer stress, however, that where resources are available every potentially viable infant should be treated.

If treatment is withheld, what alternative care is given?

> We believe that all infants deserve respect and treatment with dignity however severe their injury, simply by virtue of their humanity.
>
> (Wyatt and Spencer 1992, p. 27)

When doctors decide not to treat a very premature newborn, it usually means that the infant will receive nursing care, but no antibiotic if an infection occurs. Wyatt and Spencer (1992) advocate tender loving care from staff and parents, with warmth, hydration and analgesia for the infant when indicated.

When all life-sustaining therapies are withdrawn, the baby's comfort is the only priority. The child will not be fed by nasogastric tube, only by mouth if demanded. With most very premature babies this issue does not arise, for most have never developed the sucking reflex. Analgesics and sedatives are routinely given, even though they could bring about an earlier death, as the primary motive is to relieve distress. There are differences of opinion, however, on whether to hydrate and/or feed the neonate.

According to Campbell (1999), those caring for the child in these circumstances often have problems over withholding feeds and fluids. They feel it is unethical to let the child fade slowly away through dehydration. Campbell's opinion is that continuing with feeding and fluids only adds to the infant's suffering and serves to prolong life unnecessarily, because their failing lungs, kidneys and heart cannot cope with continued fluid intake. Continuing hydration overloads their immature systems, so by discontinuing the treatment, the infant is kept more comfortable: secretions in the lungs and throat are reduced and so breathing becomes less arduous and the risk of choking is decreased.

Wyatt and Spencer (1992), on the other hand, believe it is not acceptable to discontinue hydration and appropriate feeding by nasogastric tube if it is thought that the child might linger and suffer a slow death. They do concede, however, that if a quick death is anticipated then it is unnecessary and 'too meddlesome' to give artificial hydration or feeding. In fact, any interventions that do not contribute to relieving the baby's distress should be avoided.

Everyone concerned with the care of the child feels it is important for a child to receive appropriate and good terminal care, ending its life in the arms of its parents wherever and whenever possible. This is just as significant an outcome as is the saving of a very sick baby, and very important from the parents' point of view.

In the case of a baby who is not expected to die immediately, the parents may wish to take the child home to die in the natural environment of a loving family. In this case, it is important for them to receive full support from nursing services and their GP, with access to emergency help if needed. Wyatt and Spencer emphasise that parents can be taught the routine feeding and care for their baby and as long as all the necessary services are in place before discharge, this arrangement might be the best solution for both child and family.

Of course, for others this could be a frightening prospect, in which case all necessary facilities should be offered to them within the hospital, so that the child may die in peace and privacy in the presence of the family.

Is the decision not to treat the same as deliberately killing?

Many ethicists argue that the decision 'not to treat' is actually evading the central issue; they say that there is no moral difference between letting the patient die and actively killing them. The intention is the same and the decision to follow that line of treatment is an active one, which they know will end in the death of the baby.

> A tragic situation arose with the birth of a newborn with Down's Syndrome and duodenal atresia. The decision was to allow the newborn to die. The parents were informed that the degree of mental retardation could not be predicted. The newborn was put in a side room and after eleven days it died. Regardless of whether we agree or disagree with the decision, a more humane approach would have been euthanasia.
>
> (Heifetz 1996, p. 167)

This is an extreme example, and hopefully rarely happens; but what of those infants for whom treatment has been withheld in a futile situation because they have multiple disabilities? Death is known to be inevitable, eventually, but in the meantime the child dies a slow and possibly a painful death. Would it be more humane to use euthanasia to end its suffering? Some would argue that the moral reasoning put forward to distinguish between 'allowing to die' and direct killing loses its force in such circumstances.

Some consider that if it has been agreed that it is in the child's best interest to be allowed to die, there should be nothing to prevent the doctor from prescribing a drug to end its life quickly and painlessly. How that decision is reached and who will make it is another matter.

Davies (2001) has grave doubts about drawing any lines below which some babies are not considered suitable for resuscitation. She is sceptical about situations which make decisions appear too 'black and white' and makes the point that every situation is unique and every baby is an individual. Decisions will always be complex, but it is the doctor's duty to make crucial judgements in difficult situations. Davies believes that drawing precise parameters will only make things worse and result in more mistakes.

Withdrawing treatment

Beginning intensive care does not necessarily mean it should be continued whatever happens. In cases like that of Hamish, parents and doctors have to face a decision about whether to withdraw treatment at a later stage when irreversible neurological damage has been inflicted. On the one hand the continuation of treatment would eventually lead to a life of much suffering, requiring constant care and at great cost to child, family and society; on the other hand, withdrawal of treatment would almost certainly lead to the baby's death.

Statistics given by the Fetus & Newborn Committee of Canada (1994), showed that 90% of preterm infants with a gestational age of 23 weeks and 65% with a gestational age of 24 weeks either died or survived with long-term neurological impairment, while 85% died following the withdrawal of artificial life support (Frader and Watchko 1997).

Practices vary from hospital to hospital. Some doctors initiate aggressive treatment for all immature infants, even those weighing less than 500 grams (1lb 2oz) because they feel that an accurate prognosis cannot be assessed at birth and so they give themselves more time to consider the next course of action. Wyatt and Spencer (1992) make the point that initiating treatment in the first instance, even when it seems futile, can be a help to the parents. Sometimes they are not convinced that the child has no chance of survival, but after a short spell in intensive care they are reassured that everything possible was done for their child. It also gives them and their family time to be with the baby and to arrange a baptism or other religious rite if they so wish. Ethically, Wyatt and Spencer justify the use of scarce resources in this instance, by arguing that the emotional benefits to the parents and family of spending a few hours in intensive care bonding with their child far outweigh any resource costs involved.

However, the decision to withdraw artificial life support is painful for all concerned. The parents (and some medical staff too) may feel that they are now abandoning this tiny baby; this is why, according to some opinions, many paediatricians feel more comfortable withholding treatment from the outset. It is precisely for this reason that in some instances the practice of selective non-treatment of some very premature babies is carried out.

What criteria are used for withdrawing life support?

The initial problems facing the extremely low birth weight baby often worsen during the first three days of life as complications set in. Immature organs cannot cope with the added pressure from artificial ventilation, so heart and lungs may collapse, or liver and kidneys may fail. It is at this point that many infants die. Campbell (1999) points out that there are signs and symptoms, which are obvious, that death will eventually occur. In these circumstances the doctor's dilemma is compounded. He/she has to assess the harms and benefits of continuing to use aggressive treatment to keep this tiny infant alive, in the faint hope that some improvement may be seen; or withdrawing life support, in the belief that everything possible has been done and that it is now in the child's best interest to be left to die in peace; or, as some like to call it, 'letting nature take its course'.

The problem for both doctors and parents is to decide at what point treatment should be withdrawn. For some, the decision to withdraw life support can be justified on the grounds that any long-term hope of survival has faded. Technology is merely prolonging the process of dying for a few more hours or days. In these circumstances it seems pointless to keep on treating the tiny infant, possibly adding to its suffering and the grief of the parents. On the other hand, some parents may question whether doctors can be absolutely certain that the child will die, and may wish to continue in the belief that 'while there is life, there is hope'. Parents may be loath to let their baby go, despite assurances that, medically, they are beyond help.

What of those babies who survive the first few days? Many start to improve around the fourth day as they begin to recover from respiratory distress syndrome. As Campbell (1999) says, the use of ventilation is of prime importance in saving the lives of premature infants. Excellent results are achieved for babies who need temporary help with respiration. Ventilators give relief until the child is able to breathe unaided. However, dilemmas arise when an infant becomes so dependent on the machine that it becomes obvious that they will never be able to cope without it.

Difficulties arise when tiny immature lungs acquire some degree of damage as a result of the very treatment that saved the baby's life. Oxygen therapy and ventilation may result in broncho-pulmonary dysplasia (BPD), which slows down the baby's rate of progress and often means that they may need to stay on the ventilator in order to stay alive. This becomes a vicious circle: the longer they stay on the ventilator, the more lung damage can be sustained, which in turn means that they will be less likely to breath unaided. This results in the baby becoming more and more dependent on the ventilator, for longer and longer periods, and this situation can go on for weeks, even months. Again this can cause ethical dilemmas for practitioners and carers: how long should this treatment be maintained? The risk of further damage to other organs becomes a greater threat the longer it continues and, in the end, the future prognosis becomes very bleak.

Campbell (1999) also emphasises that ventilators can be painful and frightening. The longer the child is kept alive the greater the chance that he/she will become responsive to what is happening. Sedatives are routinely administered to relieve any pain or stress the baby may experience, but they will also dull the baby's awareness. In this sort of clinical situation, it is extremely difficult to pick up the child and cuddle or reassure them, so they become emotionally and socially isolated.

Other complications that may arise after a few days involve intracerebral haemorrhage. Some babies may have a slight bleed into the brain at the very beginning of treatment, causing minimal damage, so treatment is continued. They may then suffer a more severe neurological trauma after a further, more extensive haemorrhage at a later date. This will mean deterioration in their condition, with the likelihood that they will survive in the long term with major mental and physical disabilities. Then the dilemma is twofold: not only does it have to be decided whether life support should be withdrawn, but what degree of disability would justify that decision.

Campbell (1999) cites another scenario that complicates the decision even more. He points out that a brain haemorrhage may occur after the baby has been taken off the ventilator and is not reliant on any intensive treatment, except artificial feeding into the stomach. As all extremely low birth weight babies have not developed the sucking reflex, due to immaturity of some of the brain functions, they are dependent on routine nasogastric feeds. If brain damage is so great that the child has little chance of living without multiple and profound disabilities, should artificial feeding be withdrawn? After all, some ethicists might say that if it is acceptable to withdraw artificial ventilation from an infant, believing it to be in its own best interests, is it not also acceptable to withdraw artificial feeding for the same reason?

In all these situations the assumption is that the withdrawal of life support from this very ill baby will, at some point in the near future, result in the child's death. However, there is another scenario that is not uncommon and is the cause of great concern within the profession and with parents. If life support is withdrawn in the hope that the baby will die peacefully, but the baby actually survives, what should be done? The intention was for the child to die after it was removed from the ventilator: should further measures be taken to hasten death? If not, parents are left with a very damaged baby, who will need a lifetime of care and never live an independent existence. Many doctors feel that selective treatment at the very beginning, immediately after birth, is the best way of avoiding such a situation. For them, babies below certain weights and gestation will not be considered for resuscitation, and aggressive treatment is withheld at the outset.

DOCTRINES

Is there a moral difference between killing and letting die?

Miller (1996) offers the following scenario. The infant in question, unlike Hamish, was not premature, but the case still serves to highlight the ethical dilemma that can arise about withdrawing and withholding treatment for very ill babies and serves to illustrate the doctrines that provide a framework for doctors' judgements.

> Baby John was born by caesarean section at term, following placental abruption. He was severely asphyxiated, required ventilation and began fitting after a few hours. After a few days his condition was assessed but he appeared to be comatose and the prognosis extremely poor. After consultation with the parents it was decided to withdraw John from the ventilator and allow him to die peacefully. This was done, but he began to breathe independently in his parents' arms. He continued to breathe on his own for several weeks, but still remained floppy and unresponsive. He was again assessed and a decision taken to remove the nasogastric tube and feed only if he cried. His parents watched him grow thinner and more dehydrated as the days went by and eventually asked if John could be given something to put him and them out of their misery.
>
> (Miller 1996, p. 131)

In medicine, it is a generally accepted principle that whilst it is sometimes ethically permissible for a doctor to allow a patient to die, it is never permissible for a doctor to kill his patient. This principle is enshrined in the doctrine of acts and omissions.

The doctrine of acts and omissions

> Actions which result in some undesirable consequences are always morally worse than inactions or failures to act that the same consequences.
>
> (Gillon 1985, p. 127)

It seems reasonable to assume that the doctors mentioned earlier in Kuhse and Singer's (1985) survey would subscribe to this viewpoint; they clearly stated that while they believed it to be acceptable practice, in the case of a severely disabled infant, to allow the child to die, they would not actively end the life of that child.

Others, with a consequentialist approach, have challenged the doctrine, believing that ethically there is no fundamental difference between killing someone and allowing them to die; the outcome is the same whatever the intention.

> The only thing of value for the consequentialist is that outcomes be as good as possible. It is irrelevant, except where it makes a difference to the outcome, whether the consequences are produced by an action or an omission.
>
> (Singleton and McLaren 1995, p. 63)

Rachels (1986) goes even further, by asserting that there is no moral difference between the states of being active or passive. He argues that if it is morally permissible to act intentionally so that a person dies, then the only question that is morally significant is how to minimise their suffering in the process. To keep a suffering patient alive, knowing that death is inevitable in the near future, is harming them more than administering a lethal injection to help them towards a more peaceful death. It could be said that there are times when killing is morally preferable to 'letting die'.

From the deontological viewpoint, the principal task of a moral person is to avoid doing wrong. There are duties and laws that are paramount and we should do our utmost to uphold these, irrespective of their consequences or outcome. For the deontologist, what matters is the moral intention of an action, not its consequences, for we cannot always be certain what any eventual outcome might be.

Nancy Davis (1993) points out that deontological constraints are often negatively formulated, so that when we say 'do not lie', it is hardly the same thing as 'tell the truth'. Neither is 'do not harm' the same as 'giving assistance to those who need help'. We can see that in principle they are not the same kind of act; it is a very different thing to avoid doing harm to someone, or to actually go to their aid if they are in trouble. In the same way, if we avoid telling a lie about someone or something, it is not the same as actually telling the truth about them, given the same set of circumstances. The actions themselves are clearly different, even though they may lead to the same consequences, or even originate from the same motives.

As Davis says, these constrains on actions are 'narrowly framed and bounded', so there is little room for conflict about what is acceptable practice and what is not. From the deontological perspective, if an individual concentrates on not doing wrong, by keeping to certain rules or codes of conduct, they will be acting morally by avoiding doing harm to anyone or anything.

If we choose not to act to prevent harm, or if someone is unintentionally harmed as a result of any permissible action, it is not seen as a violation of deontological principles. Responsibility is not for what can be foreseen, but for what is intended.

The doctrine of acts and omissions is closely bound within this narrow framework and upholds the principle of 'doing no harm', as enshrined within the Hippocratic Oath: 'above all, do no harm'. If a doctor omits to act and so allows a patient to die, the deontologist claims that he/she is only 'allowing nature to take its course'.

> When one permits death by not continuing therapy, the harm that is done is by nature acting.
>
> (Collins 1968, p. 390)

The doctor is not actually harming the patient, but neither is he actively seeking to keep the patient alive, by administering drugs or therapy. The important principle here seems to be that the doctor is not causally responsible for the death of the patient. In the case of Hamish, the doctor could claim that the withdrawal of intensive treatment was not an act of deliberate killing on his part, but an attempt to alleviate his pain; the primary cause of his death was the complications directly associated with his very premature birth.

However, the point that many ethicists would make is that when the doctor decides not to give a life-saving drug, thereby 'allowing nature to take its course', his actual intention in making that decision is that the child will die.

This point is tellingly illustrated in the famous case of Dr Leonard Arthur, which I have outlined in the section in this book on the law. He prescribed massive doses of sedatives to a baby with Down's Syndrome, with the intention that the child would not live, because the parents had made it clear that they did not wish to keep the child. One of the witnesses, a Dr Dunn, speaking in defence of Dr Arthur's actions said:

> ...no paediatrician takes life, but we do accept that allowing babies to die is in the baby's interest at times.
>
> (Mason and McCall Smith 1999, p. 368)

Dr Dunn and other members of the profession made it very clear that this was normal and acceptable practice in neonatal units at that time. The difference between this case and the dilemma facing doctors in the case of Hamish was that the condition of the baby with Down's Syndrome was not critical; in fact, he appeared to be otherwise quite healthy.

McNaughton (1989) suggests that the morally significant distinction between acts and omissions is often consistent with 'planned and unplanned' consequences; omissions can be just as much part of one's purpose or intention as a positive act. Kuhse and Singer tellingly illustrate this point:

> A baby is born with spina bifida and doctors decide that it is in the child's best interest not to treat. Eventually, after a few days, the child develops a chest infection, but in the circumstances no antibiotics are given, so he dies.
>
> (Kuhse and Singer 1985, p. 80)

From the deontological view, nature has taken its course and death has occurred as a result. The doctors obeyed the principle of not acting to harm the child; but neither did they do anything to prevent its death.

Kuhse and Singer (1985) are adamant in their view that because the means of saving the child (antibiotics) were available, and the doctor chose not to use them, that omission was in fact a causal factor in the child's death. Therefore this action was just as morally wrong as if they had deliberately and actively killed the child. If the child had been an otherwise healthy child, then the same action on the part of the doctors would have been seen as negligence and as a consequence could have carried serious charges.

The distinction between planned and unplanned consequences forms the basis of the doctrine of double effect, according to McNaughton (1989).

The doctrine of double effect

> It is always wrong intentionally to do a bad act for the sake of good consequences that will ensue, but it may be permissible to do a good act in the knowledge that bad consequences will ensue.
>
> (Glover 1977, p. 86)

The doctrine of double effect emphasises the difference between the *intended* and *foreseen* consequences of an action.

Gillon (1985) points out that it was Aquinas who showed the need to define conditions where sometimes it could be morally legitimate to cause or permit evil in pursuit of good. Roman Catholic theology states that it is morally wrong to *directly intend* the death of an innocent person, for whatever motive. However, it may be permissible to perform an act that may be *foreseen* to have bad consequences, but whose *intended* consequences are only good.

> An action which has a good objective may be performed, despite the fact that the objective can only be achieved at the expense of a coincident harmful effect.
>
> (Mason and McCall Smith 1999, p. 437)

The good effects of any action must outweigh the bad. The problem is, as Mason and McCall (1999) point out, that decisions about harms and benefits may well involve value judgements. On what basis are relative harms and benefits evaluated? Who is in a position to judge the whole picture?

> A pregnant woman is diagnosed with cancer of the uterus and in order to save her life it is necessary to perform a hysterectomy. In the process, the foetus will certainly be killed.
>
> (Glover 1977, p. 87)

The doctrine of double effect would justify the action: the surgeon's *intention* when performing the surgery was to save the life of the mother; the death of the foetus was a *foreseen* but unintended side effect of that action. However, if the surgeon injected a substance into the uterus to kill the child first, this would be seen as an intentional act to harm an innocent life; killing, rather than allowing to die.

Consider the following situation. A doctor increases pain-killing medication for a dying patient, knowing that this may well shorten the life of that person. The *intention* is to alleviate pain, not to cause death, even though the consequences are almost certainly *foreseen*. However, Mason and McCall (1999) emphasise that it would be quite a different matter to administer large doses of the same drug to another patient who is also in great pain, but is expected to have a reasonable chance of recovery.

Implications for neonatal intensive care

If we return to the plight of Hamish for a moment, we can see the relevance of this doctrine in the context of caring for very premature babies. Decisions were made in the first minutes after his precipitous birth to treat him by using invasive and artificial methods to save and prolong his life. He is kept alive only because of this equipment, but it is now known that he has been profoundly damaged in the process and that further aggressive therapy will not improve his prognosis and only cause him more suffering. What is to be done in the circumstances? Would the withdrawal of life support mean that those responsible for turning off the machines were guilty of infanticide, or are there other issues to be considered?

The decision to withdraw artificial life support from Hamish could be supported within the doctrine of double effect, by arguing that the *intention* of this act was to ease further suffering and distress for the baby, and in his best interests. His death may have been *foreseen* as a consequence of the action, but was not the primary motive.

Ordinary and extraordinary means

> The good of saving life is morally obligatory only if its pursuit is not excessively burdensome or disproportionate in relation to the expected benefits.
>
> (Gillon 1985, p. 141)

This is another Roman Catholic doctrine that allows treatment to be withheld from a patient, when it will not significantly improve the patient's condition or prolong their life, and is likely to cause more harm than respite. The definition of what 'extraordinary' treatment means can vary; what might be classed as ordinary in one set of circumstances, could be considered as extraordinary in another. In the case of the baby with spina bifida mentioned previously, the medical judgement was that the child's disabilities were such that, in the circumstances, prescribing antibiotics would be inappropriate and 'extraordinary' treatment, whereas had the child not been born with a disability, the treatment would have been deemed appropriate and necessary.

In practice this doctrine can prove difficult to apply: for some it could mean the withdrawal of antibiotics or ventilation, or decisions against performing surgery. Wells (1989) indicates that the doctrine is used more for determining the non-treatment of patients in hopeless situations; it is particularly relevant to selective treatment in neonatal intensive care. In the case of Hamish and others like him who are kept alive by artificial means, the doctrine of ordinary and extraordinary means is very much a reality. Withholding or withdrawing treatment from such infants may be seen as saving them from a life 'not worth living'; such decisions would, however, have to be made after careful evaluation of each individual case.

Others might argue the case for the withdrawal of nutrition in extreme situations. Consider this scenario: a child is withdrawn from the ventilator, in the belief that death will shortly follow. Against all expectations he continues to live, breathing unaided. His prognosis is still very poor and his expected quality of life minimal when judged by 'normal' standards. What kind of treatment should the infant now be given? Is he to continue being fed and hydrated, or can the withdrawal of nutrition be justified on the grounds that in this situation it is considered an 'extraordinary' means of treatment? After all, the baby's death had been anticipated and planned, and previous decisions were based on the belief that the child's life was too burdensome to bear; the prognosis has not changed, but the child has continued to live.

In such extreme cases, some Dutch paediatricians have advocated prescribing medication to actively bring about the death of such a baby. In other words, they advocate the practice of active euthanasia on the grounds that by keeping the child alive they are permitting more suffering and harm; therefore morally it is better to end the child's distress sooner rather than later. The ethical issues involved with euthanasia are discussed later in this section.

Guidelines for paediatricians on withholding and withdrawing treatment

The Ethics Advisory Committee believe that there is no moral distinction between the withholding and withdrawal of life-saving treatment, given the same ethical objective, but emphasise that in either case, it does not mean that an infant should receive no care at all. They recommend that decisions should be made by experienced senior staff and that neonates should almost always be resuscitated, particularly if there has been no prior discussion.

Babies born at 23 weeks' gestation or less should not be resuscitated when parents accept the doctor's prognosis that the child is severely neurologically damaged and that a prolonged stay in intensive care would be futile.

Artificial ventilation should be withdrawn from a child who has subsequently been found to be suffering profound brain damage.

The duty of care is not an absolute duty to preserve life by all means. There is no obligation to provide life sustaining treatment if its use is inconsistent with the aims and objectives of an appropriate treatment plan, or if the burdens of the treatment outweigh the benefits to the patient. This is referred to as the 'no purpose' situation.

A redirection of management from life-sustaining treatment to palliation represents a change in beneficial aims and objectives, and does not constitute a withdrawal of care.

A distinction is drawn between treatment of the dying patient and euthanasia. When a dying patient is receiving palliative care, the underlying cause of death is the disease process. In euthanasia, the cause of death is the intended lethal action.

It follows that the use of medication and other treatments that may incidentally hasten death may be justified if the primary aim is to relieve suffering. The Committee does not support the concept of active euthanasia.

The Committee accepts that there are circumstances when the continuation of active medical interventions in an otherwise futile situation will do nothing more than cause suffering to the child. It then seems more appropriate for palliative care to be offered as an alternative, providing support and comfort for both child and family in this distressing situation. The Committee's decisions are based on three key principles:

1. The duty of care and the partnership of care

The first duty is to sustain life; the second is to restore health. If restoration of health is not possible, then the duty is to comfort, cherish and prevent pain and suffering.

2. The legal duty

Any practice or treatment given with the primary intention of causing death is unlawful.

3. Respect for children's rights

The second two points, referring to the legal implications, are covered in Section 2 of this book.

12

Abortion, infanticide and neonaticide

> A woman can terminate a perfectly healthy pregnancy by abortion at 24 weeks and that is legal. Nature can terminate a problem pregnancy by miscarriage at 24 weeks and the baby must be saved at all costs; anything less is illegal and immoral.
>
> (A quote from Peggy Stinson's diary. Singer 1996, p. 84)

The very fact that it is now possible to save infants born before the 24th week of pregnancy has created another medical dilemma, illustrated in the above quote: What, if any, is the moral difference between a late abortion and a premature baby born with the same gestational age?

Consider the case of an American couple, Peggy and Robert Stinson.

> The Stinsons were forced to contemplate a late abortion, 24 weeks into the pregnancy, because of a placenta praevia, which was threatening to detach from the uterus and cause danger to the lives of both mother and child. They were also told that if the baby did survive there was a chance that it could be seriously damaged. They were assured that although it was late in the pregnancy an abortion could be performed safely and legally under American law.
>
> However, before they had come to a definite decision, Peggy started premature labour and gave birth to a baby boy between 24 and 25 weeks of pregnancy. It was doubtful whether he would survive; even if he did, there was a high risk of brain damage. The Stinsons requested that there should be no medical intervention to save their baby, but the paediatrician threatened court action if they did not give consent for aggressive treatment. Artificial respiration was started, but it soon became apparent that the baby had suffered injury and even if he did live he would be disabled.

Peggy was perplexed by the paradox of a situation whereby a neonatal special care unit is saving very premature babies at less than 24 weeks' gestation at any cost, while in the same hospital another department is aborting perfectly healthy foetuses of the same gestational age. If it is morally and legally acceptable for a child to be aborted at a certain point in gestation, why should it be morally obligatory to save the life of another child, born at the same point of gestation, who has spontaneously aborted?

Tooley (1972) suggests that because the topic of infanticide raises strong emotions and is almost a taboo subject for most people, we fight shy of ever getting to grips with the really thorny issues involved in this area and so fail to address them rationally. Nevertheless, these difficult ethical questions need to be addressed. The boundaries have been pushed back, beyond the legal limit for viability, and the challenge is whether any arguments can be presented to show that infanticide is morally wrong. If it is deemed legally permissible for a woman to request an abortion to kill a malformed foetus of 23 weeks' gestation, why are we not allowed to do the same to an infant who has been born very prematurely and suffered profound mental and physical injuries in the process? Is there a moral difference between the two? It does seem irrational to argue the case for one and then deny the case for the other.

If, then, there is no moral difference between these acts, why do most people find the notion of abortion quite tolerable but the notion of infanticide so abhorrent? Heifetz (1996) believes that the act of abortion is more readily accepted in society because of the limited opportunity to bond with the child before birth. Whilst we may accept a decision to abort an unwanted 23-week foetus, to withhold treatment of a 23-week premature infant, whose birth has been eagerly awaited, and whose parents have already touched and held him, is quite a different matter, even though the baby may have suffered irreversible brain trauma. The difference, Heifetz believes, is not based on reason, but on an intense sorrow at the thought of a newborn's death, because the parents have already begun to bond with the child.

Paradoxically, most aborted foetuses, who are not protected in law, would have become normal healthy babies had they continued in the womb, while those spontaneously aborted and profoundly impaired infants have full legal protection.

INFANTICIDE: A HISTORICAL AND CULTURAL PERSPECTIVE

Most people would prefer to raise children who do not suffer from gross deformities or from severe physical emotional or intellectual handicaps. If it could be shown that there is no moral objection to infanticide the happiness of society could be significantly and justifiably increased.

(Tooley 1972, p. 39)

Infanticide undoubtedly is murder, since the displeasure of the law is not concerned with ages, but with a breach to the human race.

(Philo, in Ferngren 1987, p. 23)

Among the many problems faced by this sort of position are the widespread and deeply felt intuitions that newborn infants are of the same moral importance as the rest of us and have the same right to life.

(Raanan Gillon 1985, p. 53)

Many cultures, in both the ancient world and today's society, have practised infanticide. Wyatt and Spencer (1992) cite the Graeco-Roman civilisations where a child's value and right to life wad based upon their future potential as a worthy citizen rather than their intrinsic value as a human being. Children born with congenital abnormalities or disease were considered to be virtually worthless and had little right to life. Wyatt and Spencer quote the Roman physician Soranus who wrote a manual of instructions for midwives in the 2nd century AD entitled 'How to recognise the Newborn that is Worth Rearing'. He described how midwives should examine and assess each newborn to ensure that they were perfectly healthy and to recognise the signs and symptoms that separated them from those infants who were not considered worth rearing. The ethics of killing defective or very ill newborn babies, by drowning or exposure to the elements, was not even an issue worthy of debate.

Nowadays the term infanticide has both a technical and a general legal meaning, according to Mason and McCall Smith (1999). In the general sense, it just means the killing of an infant. However, under English law, the meaning is confined to the killing of a child under the age of 12 months, by its mother, and is enshrined in the Infanticide Act 1938. It is said that babies less than a year old are four times more likely to be killed than any other group. The 1938 Act, which distinguishes the crime of infanticide from that of murder, recognises that it is not uncommon for women to suffer mental instability in the months following childbirth (including postnatal depression, puerperal psychosis, or Munchausen's Syndrome by proxy). In these circumstances a mother who has killed her own child is dealt with sympathetically by the courts, as long as she is willing to admit her guilt.

However, as Mason and McCall Smith (1999) point out, studies on the subject of infanticide show that just over a quarter of infant deaths caused by the mother were not due to any of the above reasons. In recent months there has been a great deal of publicity around a few cases of women who have been found guilty of murdering their young offspring and sentenced to life imprisonment. In all cases, these mothers have refused to plead guilty, maintaining that the child died from sudden infant death syndrome, or 'cot death'.

Professor Rupert Risdon, a histopathologist at Great Ormond Street Hospital, believes that the crime of infanticide is far more widespread than anyone realises:

> A young baby is very vulnerable and easy to kill without leaving any signs. People can't get their heads around the notion of a mother smothering her child; but if you live in the world I do, you know that it goes on a lot.
>
> (Independent on Sunday, 21st April 2002, p. 19)

NEONATICIDE

In law, the deliberate killing of any human being is murder; the killing of a multiply disabled baby is no exception. Brazier (1992) tells us that immediately the child has an independent existence from its mother (that is, when it has independent circulation and possibly before the placenta has been fully expelled from the mother), the law protects him.

However, there are those who believe that the treatment of damaged neonates raises certain issues that are separate from those surrounding the treatment of damaged or sick adults. Brazier points out that the plight of the baby differs from that of someone who has become severely disabled later in life, as a result of injury or illness. The child has never known, and will never know, any other existence. They have no expectations or appreciation of what life without disabilities could be. There seems to have been a shift in the climate of opinion within the medical profession, which means, for some, that the life of the damaged neonate has a lesser value than the life of someone older; and just as it is permissible to terminate the life of a damaged foetus, so it should be with the life of a profoundly damaged neonate.

What are the reasons for this shift of opinion? Firstly, paediatricians are increasingly aware of the long term damage which can be inflicted on very premature babies who are subjected to long periods of aggressive treatment to save their lives. Secondly, Section 37 of the Human Fertilisation and Embryology Act now permits damaged foetuses to be aborted right up to the end of pregnancy. So, it is difficult to follow the logic that allows the destruction of a damaged life up to 40 weeks' gestation, while at the same time actively striving to save babies whose disability was not detected until birth.

In addition, the sanctity of life principle has been eroded and challenged by the view that the real value of life is to be found in its quality and how much it contributes to the whole of society, rather than in its intrinsic worth. Although there are those who will argue forcefully against such ideas, quality of life considerations do seem to be gaining ground when difficult dilemmas occur in the neonatal unit.

Proposals have been made for specific legislation about the practice of neonaticide, the grounds for which, according to Brazier (1992), are as follows:

1. The law needs clarification. Doctors need a safeguard that would protect them from having to face test cases in the courts (like the case of Dr Leonard Arthur, who was charged with the murder of a baby with Down's Syndrome).
2. The law should be more ready to allow doctors to withhold treatment from children whose quality of life is known to be very poor if parents agree with the decision.
3. The law should enable active measures to be taken to end the life of a child rather than allow it to suffer a lingering and painful death.

The response by the medical profession to such proposals has not been enthusiastic; in some circles it has been overtly hostile.

The actual proposals for legislation are outlined in this book, in the section entitled The Legal Framework.

EUTHANASIA

The term euthanasia is derived from the Greek 'eu' meaning 'good' and 'thanatos' meaning 'death'. It is commonly used to refer to an action, motivated by mercy, of deliberately bringing about death in a humane or painless way in order to prevent or reduce any further suffering for an individual.

- Active euthanasia (or 'mercy killing') is when a person actively and directly causes death.
- Passive euthanasia is when the death is caused by a failure to intervene to prolong life. It is referred to in medicine as the withdrawing or withholding of life-supporting mechanisms.
- Voluntary euthanasia is administered at the patient's request. Obviously this is irrelevant in the case of the neonate, who has no capacity for knowing or expressing their wishes.
- Involuntary euthanasia or non-voluntary euthanasia is paternalistically instigated, the primary motive being to promote the patient's best interests.

It is a widely acknowledged fact that passive neonatal euthanasia has been practised and condoned for many years, although the ethical arguments justifying the custom are seldom clear. As we have seen earlier, the principle of paternalism motivated by beneficence and non-maleficence often governs the doctor's actions in order to do the best for his patients. In the normal doctor-patient relationship, when the patient is competent and autonomous, the principle of autonomy will outweigh any paternalistic approach. For the paediatrician in the neonatal unit, the principles of beneficence and non-maleficence will outweigh the principle of autonomy. Alongside these is the principle of justice, which states that the infant should be treated in exactly the same way that any other child in the same circumstances would be treated, and that the rights of the child are protected at all times. In the case of the very premature and damaged infant, many people see the parental views as decisive. The parents become the channel through which the baby accepts or rejects treatment, and should have the final say in decision making.

Parents and practitioners are called upon to make crucial

decisions in a situation when the life of a critically ill newborn is at stake. The ethical dilemmas are complex and the four principles of autonomy, beneficence, non-maleficence and justice may each sustain arguments to support various, even opposing, options for treatment.

Can neonatal euthanasia ever be justified?

There are situations where some paediatricians would consider *active* neonatal euthanasia morally justifiable, sometimes even morally obligatory. Pence (1995) cites Goldman as saying that death is only an evil if the continuation of a patient's life would be of benefit to that patient. When a death is 'good', killing cannot be a harm and therefore is not unethical.

> A premature baby was saved and kept alive by mechanical means, but is now suffering profound neurological damage, leaving it seriously mentally and physically disabled. The prognosis is so bleak that parents and doctors decide that in the best interests of the child it would be better to withdraw treatment and allow the child to die peacefully. Despite this the baby continues to breathe on its own.

> An infant is born with such severe congenital abnormalities that attempts at surgery are thought to be futile and so withheld, but the child continues to survive.

In such extreme circumstances as these, it is argued that if the future quality of life for the child and its family are so awful in every respect, the doctor should be allowed, as an 'act of mercy', to end the life of the child. Those who concur with this view believe that active euthanasia in the newborn, or neonaticide, is the most humane answer to a devastating situation. Englehardt (1975) introduced the concept of 'injury of continued existence', where, in some situations, within the principle of non-maleficence, it is morally preferable to allow death:

> The concept of injury for continuance of existence, the proposed analogue of the concept of tort for wrongful life can be of negative value, such that the medical maxim 'primum non nocere' (first do no harm) would require not sustaining life.
>
> (Englehardt 1975, p. 87)

Looking at it from this perspective, if the burdens outweigh the benefits and when all avenues have been explored, allowing a seriously ill neonate to die does not violate the doctor's obligation of non-maleficence.

Inevitably, other paediatricians hold strong opposing views. They feel that although it is justifiable for doctors to withhold treatment if they believe it is harming rather than benefiting the baby, actively taking steps to end the baby's life can never be morally justified. For them, the practice of medicine is about the preservation of life not its destruction. These practitioners would subscribe to the view that it is better to allow 'nature to take its course' and so opt for non-treatment; not intervening if infections or other life-threatening conditions arise.

Whatever their stance on this issue, whichever side of the ethical debate they stand, in the end all doctors know that to take active steps to end the life of any patient, whether they are very old or very young, is against the law. Nevertheless, the debate about whether there is a moral difference between omitting to act, knowing that by doing so the patient will surely die, and taking active steps to end life, is one that will not go away.

13

Life and death decisions: who should make them?

PARENTS ARE IN THE BEST POSITION TO DECIDE

Decisions about whether to withdraw treatment from a very sick baby are, by their very nature, heart-rending for all concerned.

Both Davies (2001) and Campbell (1999) believe that when the prognosis is uncertain or when it looks very bleak, and when doctors are wondering about whether to resuscitate or continue aggressive treatment, the parents should be the primary decision-makers. If medical staff had all the answers, and could give an accurate prognosis, then they should be in a position to make crucial decisions. Doctors may offer advice and guidance after they have given parents all the facts about their child's diagnosis and prognosis, but when parents and doctors are both in the same situation and nobody knows for certain what the future holds, then parents should be left to face the realities that confront them and make an informed decision about what treatment their child should receive. Of course, it should be emphasised that in order to make their agonising decision, the parents do need to be fully informed about their baby's condition.

Miller (1996) and Walters (1986) see parents as the rightful decision makers; they are responsible for most decisions about their children's lives and upbringing; it seems contradictory that they should be denied this right immediately after birth. They are the ones who will be left to rear the child for as long as they or it lives, and to live with the difficulties which life will certainly bring.

Only ten years ago, parents played little part in the decision-making process about the withholding or withdrawing of treatment for their baby, because it was thought that the stress they were suffering, and their lack of understanding about the clinical diagnosis, made their judgement suspect. Nowadays the situation has moved on and parents are encouraged to take a more active role in decision making.

If parents decide, after listening to advice, that they wish therapy to continue, then their wishes should be honoured; although Campbell (1999) does insist that the doctor should tactfully continue to promote his/her own views.

There may be strong cultural, religious, family and community ties that will have a bearing on the parents' choice. They may wish to offer their baby every possible chance of life, whatever the cost, knowing that this may mean a lifetime of caring for a profoundly disabled child. Or, on the other hand, they could be influenced by the grim statistics, therefore choosing to discontinue life support and allowing the child to die without further suffering. Whatever their choice, and however they reach their decision, as long as they are fully informed and truly believe that they are acting in the best interests of their child, then the final decision must rest with the parents.

Doctors, nurses and health care workers in the field all have a personal opinion about the correct course of action. Some will feel it wrong to continue what they feel is futile treatment. Others will presume that the sanctity of life argument means that it would be wrong to discontinue life support. Everybody has their own personal beliefs and baggage. But it is wrong for anyone, whether medically trained or not, to believe that they know what is best for another family in this particular circumstance. It is natural for anyone to wonder what we would do in the same circumstances, but it would be wrong for the parents to be judged on whatever decision they make, if that decision is not in accord with our own.

> When the best path is unclear, fully informed parents are the best decision-makers. No one is closer to that baby, in blood, body and spirit than the mother and father. Their best guess is the best one of all. No one else can decide for his or her baby as carefully, thoughtfully, purposefully and solemnly as they do. No one else can be more agonised, calculating and soul-searching. This is a decision that must be made with the mind, gut and heart. Your own baby would want you to make this decision, not strangers.
>
> (Deborah Davies 1999, p. 1)

Of course it may be that parents are too emotionally distressed after the birth to make such crucial decisions; they may not feel ready to take the full responsibility for deciding whether their child lives or dies. It may be that they cannot face a lifetime of guilt: letting the baby go now would mean forever agonising and wondering whether they did the right thing.

> The despair I felt at that moment was bottomless... because I felt the whole responsibility had been heaped onto me and I could not see how I could make that decision and go on living with myself.
>
> (Miller 1996, p. 130)

PARENTS ARE NOT IN THE BEST POSITION TO DECIDE

Miller (1996) argues that parents may not necessarily be in the best position to make crucial decisions at this time for a number of reasons. They may not, for example, be able to grasp the degree of handicap anticipated and what that might mean for the child. She also questions whether it is right for parents to be left feeling that the burden of responsibility for making decisions about their child's life or death lies solely with them. Although in normal circumstances parents are considered responsible for decisions affecting their children, in extreme cases they may not be in a fit state to make critical judgements about appropriate treatment.

Tyson (1995) too, believes that there are situations when parents should not be involved in decisions about the child's treatment. He cites the American view that when a premature baby is born, if the evidence is strong and the cost is judged to be acceptable, then treatment is mandatory; the doctor is obliged to administer neonatal intensive care. Parents have no right to ask that treatment be withheld. He clarifies this by citing the example of an infant born at 31 weeks' gestation, birth weight 1500 grams (3lb 8oz), with respiratory distress syndrome. If the resources within the hospital are not adequate, the infant should be transferred to another unit where appropriate treatment is available. However, it would be unreasonable to begin intensive treatment if there is little or no evidence that the baby would benefit and when the expected value of that care would not justify the costs; the type of infant he cites in this case is one weighing 250 grams (9oz), born at 20 weeks, with a slow heart rate. In this situation parents would not participate in decision making and would have no right to demand neonatal intensive care, and physicians ought not to administer neonatal intensive care.

Nevertheless, Tyson does advocate that parents have a right to be involved in decision making whenever neonatal intensive care is optional or investigational. However, if parents would like more time to think about options, the doctor should be allowed the freedom to initiate treatment in the meantime.

It has been suggested that preparation during pregnancy for the possibility of a premature birth and its complications, could help both parents and neonatologists to understand each other's problems and come to some agreement on parental preferences and appropriate treatments should such a situation arise.

Sometimes, however, there are practical issues that may cause problems in actually achieving this aim. When decisions have to be made quickly about withholding or beginning treatment (during labour, or shortly after delivery) the mother may not be in a physical or mental condition to take on board the full implications of what is being said to her. She may be ill, through some complication due to pregnancy and birth; she may be heavily sedated, or recovering from a caesarean section; the father may be unavailable. Sometimes the baby needs to be moved to another unit, miles away, and parents cannot be contacted when immediate intervention is needed. Even during the days and weeks following the birth some doctors claim that 'adequately' or 'fully' informed consent may be impossible, even when they have given the parents all relevant information. Almost certainly both parents will be suffering significant emotional stress, which may hinder their capacity to think clearly; they may be very young and too immature to take on board the significance or severity of the child's condition, or they may not have the mental ability to understand what is being said.

SUBSTITUTED JUDGEMENT

> To follow the regime that one assumes the patient him/herself would have opted for if given the chance.
>
> (Mason and McCall Smith 1999, p. 374)

Mason and McCall Smith (1999) describe the concept of 'substituted judgement' as one that enables decision makers to eliminate what they describe as the hypocrisy surrounding 'best interests' judgements, which are supposedly in the sole interests of the patient, yet are often tempered by considerations about the family's needs and sometimes by resource issues. These interests should not be condemned as irrelevant: they are often very pertinent to the case in question. However, according to Mason and McCall Smith, by using substituted judgement decision-makers are able to quite legitimately take all these things into account. Any competent patient who opts for non-treatment will have made their choice by considering some or all of these elements. Therefore it is perfectly reasonable to incorporate them into any substituted judgement made on behalf of an incompetent patient or, as in this case, an extremely premature infant.

The theory of substituted judgement involves putting ourselves in the place of the child, and asking ourselves fundamental questions: Would we would want the chance to live at any cost, despite agonizing physical disabilities, without any chance of improvement? Or would we consider death preferable to the prospect of a lifetime of pain, disability and dependence on others for every need?

Obviously, it is impossible for us to know what any baby would want to do, but we do know that most people tend to share the views of their family on many issues. Mason and McCall Smith believe that when deciding what is in the best interests of the child, we should think in terms of *'best interests'* as against *'no interests'*. If a patient is in great pain, death could be thought of as a 'blessed release' and therefore in their best interests. However, an incompetent patient, like the very premature baby with serious and permanent neurological damage, who has no hope of ever developing any awareness of self or others, they can have no interest in whether they live or die. It is in these cases where substituted judgement becomes relevant.

So the theory of substituted judgement means that although the child cannot and will never have a view on the subject, owing to its age and profound disability, the parents can rightly make a decision for the child in the knowledge that they are acting in a way that has the child's best interests at heart and accords with their own shared values. They can feel reassured that if the child were capable of making a decision, then it would be the one that they have chosen.

Some people are very clear from the beginning what their

decision will be. Some will urge doctors to do everything possible to keep the child alive, whatever the future may hold. They are prepared to face any future problems, however devastating, and deal with issues as they arise. Others feel that if the prognosis is bleak, they should not allow their child to suffer unnecessarily and perhaps face a lifetime of pain and indignity. Like those parents we have quoted, they may request that the baby be withdrawn from intensive treatment, to die in peace. Both views are legitimate in what is an agonising and unenviable crisis.

For many other loving parents, knowing the facts and the different points of view only makes the decision all the more heart-rending, especially if they have a difference of opinion. Campbell (1999) suggests that it is the child's best interests that should be considered at all times; but he makes the point that they should not, indeed cannot, be separated from the interests of the family. The effects of a lifelong commitment to an individual with profound and multiple disabilities must be clear to the parents and other family members.

Robertson (1998) questions the validity of substituted judgement and is sceptical of the claim that these 'proxy judgements' can ever be neutral, claiming that doctors and parents may be influenced by their own interests rather than solely by the interests of the child. Even a so-called neutral proxy may have problems with egocentricity and knowing what is in another's mind. When someone makes a proxy judgement, we are told that they are basing their assumptions on what any ordinary, reasonable person would think in the circumstances. For Robertson, this is entirely the wrong way of looking at this particular issue. For him, proxy judgements have the capacity for wide margins of error. Clinical judgements about future prospects and prognoses are not infallible and may still be wide of the mark in many cases. Quality of life decisions should only be applied in those cases where it is known that the child's condition is incompatible with life or where profound mental impairment is a certainty. It is inappropriate to assume that a person would prefer death to a life of pain, suffering and social isolation. The point that Robertson makes is that someone who has never known a life of health, happiness and fulfilment will never be in a position to suffer their loss in the same way as someone who has already experienced and enjoyed them. Someone who has indeed known their advantages, (in other words a 'reasonable person') may indeed prefer death to the prospect of living the rest of their lives with such disabilities, but it does not follow that the person who has never experienced them would feel the same. For them, life itself may be of sufficient value to make it worth living. Do we have the right to deny them this chance of life, albeit one which others of us may not be prepared to accept for ourselves?

In order to avoid any biased decisions some people believe that the only way to decide the right course of action is to rely on the judgement of an ethics committee. They feel that this is the best means of ensuring the baby's best interests and that it can help resolve conflicting views about treatment between professionals. This method would probably reduce the part played by parents in the decision-making process, which is why others question the role of formal committee decisions about such crucial issues.

On balance, most professionals and parents feel the informal discussions that take place between all those who have an interest in the child's welfare, at each stage of the infant's treatment, are the most beneficial and acceptable. The important factor is that discussions are open and informative, so that all parties feel free to voice their concerns and opinions in an accepting and understanding environment.

PATERNALISM AND PARENTAL AUTONOMY

In the very delicate area of neonatal intensive care, the relationship between parents and doctors is crucial. The sophisticated technology used in treatment can make parents feel helpless and inadequate when asked to make decisions or to give their consent for further medication. Treatments and procedures that health care workers see as routine in their daily work with very ill babies can seem frightening to lay people who are in no position to understand what is going on. Therefore communication between doctors and parents is vital. It is in this context that problems arising from paternalism versus autonomy, truthfulness and informed consent sometimes emerge.

How much should parents be told and how much can they be expected to understand? Brindle and Roseley (1997) point to a Mencap survey of 1000 families with special needs children under the age of eleven and found that the majority were very unhappy about the treatment they received from their doctors. Only 23% of the families questioned said they felt the doctors were really knowledgeable about the problems surrounding mental handicap and 33% were unhappy with the ways the news was broken to them; they were either alone or given very little support at the time.

One young mother would certainly agree with this; I shall call her Judith. This is what she told me about her memories surrounding the birth of her second child; they serve to highlight the ethical problems that can arise when parental rights and autonomy conflict with the paternalistic attitude of medical staff.

> It was immediately obvious there were physical disabilities with the baby's legs and feet, but it soon became obvious that there were also other abnormalities involving kidney and digestive tract. He had breathing problems due to fits in the early days, leaving him with brain damage and severe learning disabilities. He is now four years old and has profound and multiple mental and physical problems.
>
> Judith described the nightmare of trying to cope with a baby who constantly screamed, had fits and vomited back his feeds, in addition to coping with the demands of her other child, a normal energetic toddler. Judith and her husband felt strongly that the support from paediatricians and hospital staff was both inadequate and at times insensitive. No one explained to her what was wrong, or why the baby had been taken away. The first comment that she was aware of was, "Never mind dear, orthopaedic surgeons can do wonders these days." This was before she had even seen her baby, who was wrapped tightly in a shawl. She remembers recoiling in horror, wondering what on earth she was going to see when she unwrapped the covers.
>
> She tells of the day when one midwife who was examining the baby's deformed feet and legs, commented "Huh, this is probably *his* fault," referring to Judith's husband.
>
> As the weeks went by and the child's condition deteriorated, Judith and her husband made their wishes known to the medical staff and social work team that they felt it in his best interests that he should be allowed to die. He was still being fed by nasogastric tube and even then he was vomiting most of his food back and they asked for it to be removed, so that he may be allowed to die 'with dignity' (Judith's words).

The result of that meeting was that the couple were informed that if they insisted on their wishes being carried out, then the medical staff would have no alternative but to make the little boy a ward of court.

The lack of information about the child's condition, and the way the news was broken to her, left Judith imagining all sorts of horrendous deformities. A flippant, throwaway remark about the cause of the disability was not only unprofessional, it was unforgivable and completely unfounded. The nurse probably forgot the comment within minutes, but for someone trying to come to terms with the birth of a very sick infant it was unforgettable.

Judith and her husband were both convinced that their baby's life was too painful to bear. To them he was obviously distressed by the constant interference of invasive procedures, and was not thriving. They believed that their rights and autonomy as parents had been severely undermined: their concerns either went unheard or were overruled by professionals who believed they knew better.

It seems that the emphasis moved from baby to mother when Judith and her husband made it known that they wanted treatment withdrawn. It was suggested that Judith had problems: she must be suffering postnatal depression and was therefore obviously not in any fit state to make rational decisions. The parents gave up their fight when they were told that there would be an application to make the child a ward of court if they continued. They were concerned that any further stress could only have a more damaging effect on the family; and they had the welfare of their other child to consider too.

Forshaw (1995) confirms the dilemma between parental autonomy and doctors' paternalism, maintaining that babies are frequently given treatment without parental consent. When this results in benefits to the child, parental rights are rarely invoked, but if it results in harm to the child then the resulting conflict may become an issue resolved only by the courts. However, the ultimate decision about treatment does lie firmly with the doctor concerned; the conflict here is seen when there is disagreement between parent and Consultant, while both claim to be acting in the child's best interests.

Similar attitudes are illustrated in an article written by another mother, Kate Sainsbury (1998) as she describes how she felt helpless to protect her newborn child from the harm of severe brain damage, because the Consultant in charge overruled her wishes. She argues that not enough weight is given to parental wishes or to the fact that they are the ones who will eventually bear the brunt of caring for the child.

There was no one to support my belief that medication had come too late and that the quality of life for my son would be so greatly impaired that the treatment was wrong. The consultant insisted on treating: 'But I give you my word that society will always care for him,' he promised.

> He had authority on his side. All I had was a passionate concern for my child and a fear that the system was condemning him to a lifetime of dependency on a state that, in reality, did not live up to the consultant's ideals.
>
> (Sainsbury 1998, p. 6)

The paediatrician described in this incident seems particularly high-handed and paternalistic in his dealings with parents. The promise, on behalf of society, to care for the child showed a complete lack of understanding of the parents' feelings and no knowledge of resource issues in today's political climate. In the circumstances, was the doctor morally right to make such a promise? For Wells (1989) the answer is unequivocal:

> There is a moral and ethical problem of the most fundamental sort involved in a system which allows complicated decisions of this nature to be made unilaterally by people who do not have to live with the consequences of their decisions.
>
> (Wells 1989, p. 198)

Both Judith and Kate Sainsbury were convinced that their child should not be allowed to continue suffering any longer. Davies (2001) confirms that from her work with bereaved parents and parents of premature babies, the predominant concern that is expressed by parents is the amount of suffering their child will endure. Whether they ultimately decide to 'let nature take its course', or whether they opt for aggressive treatment, the primary concern is not the prospect of living with a severely disabled child, but how much pain and suffering the child would have to bear, both immediately and in the future.

According to Wells' (1989) survey of mothers of severely disabled young adults, two thirds wished in retrospect that they had had an abortion, while twelve out of fifteen thought it would have been better for the babies to have been allowed to die peacefully rather than be saved by aggressive intervention.

Tyson (1995) quotes Silverman in this situation. He argues for balancing the interests of the infant, the family and society:

> Parents of a badly damaged baby often resent the implied demand that their family is required to pass a 'sacrifice test' to satisfy the moral expectations of those who do not have to live, day by day, with the consequences of diffuse idealism. It is easy, some parents say, to demand prolongation of each and every new life that requires none of one's own ... resources to maintain that life later.
>
> (Tyson 1995, p. 4)

The parents of one such premature infant said:

> As Andrew's parents we had a heightened sense of his suffering. Also we feared the prospect of having to care for the rest of our lives for a pathetically handicapped and retarded child. If this is considered less than noble, what then is the appropriate label for the willingness to apply the latest experimental technology to salvage such a high risk child and then hand him over to the life long care of someone else?
> (Stinson 1981, p. 18)

This statement clearly challenges the claim made by the doctor described by Sainsbury (1998) that society would care for the child. These parents clearly felt that the burden of responsibility would be theirs and they were not prepared for such a sacrifice. They questioned the paternalism shown by the doctor who thought he knew what was best for them and their offspring.

Mutch (1997) agrees that doctors can sometimes unwittingly contribute to a sense of powerlessness, by excluding parents from discussions and withholding information. Forshaw (1995) maintains that apart from other problems it can lead to an over-dependence on the medical team, because parents are expected to make so little contribution to the decision-making process that they never acquire enough knowledge or skills to feel confident enough to take over the care of the baby. This view seems to be confirmed by studies undertaken by Cunningham and Davis (1985) who found that parents' previous experience and interpretation of life does not necessarily prepare them for the news of their child's disability and they are left with a sense of guilt and despair that they are powerless to do anything to change things. This sense of despair is magnified if they feel that doctors are not being entirely honest with them, or that they are not being given enough information to make any meaningful contribution to decisions about their child's future. Therefore their wishes and opinions are of little value.

TRUTH TELLING AND INFORMED CONSENT

When doctors and family disagree or clash about treatment or consent to treatment the situation can become very unpleasant (Sarah Boseley 2001). In 1997 a disagreement arose between the parents of two premature babies, one of whom died. The parents claimed that the baby had been part of a trial led by David Southall, a leading neonatologist, practising in a hospital in the

Midlands. The parents claimed that they had not been told the truth about the treatment in neonatal intensive care and had not consented to any such treatment on their babies.

The trials were on a new type of ventilator machine called CNEP (continuous negative extrathoracic pressure), which is similar to an iron lung, and in which babies were placed to help expand their chest and help them breathe more easily. This was achieved by changing pressure inside the machine.

The mother of these babies claimed that she had no idea at the time that the children were involved in trials until it was confirmed that Sophie had cerebral palsy after suffering a brain haemorrhage. She said that at the time she had been led to believe that the child had benefited from the latest treatment and that she only discovered that it was 'experimental' at a later date.

The hospital trust stated that a consent form was signed. The mother said that she was shown a form, but did not remember signing it, adding that even if she did sign it, she had no idea what she was signing for.

The Consultant was suspended from duty pending an enquiry into allegations that consent forms had been forged in order to obtain infants for dubious research purposes. A campaign began in the press. The case evoked strong feelings on both sides. The Consultant was described as brilliant, caring, courageous and passionate about his work with premature infants by his supporters; many of whom were parents of babies he had saved. His accusers said that he was reckless and single minded in the pursuit of his own interests.

The enquiry took two years, generating much controversy; it eventually found in David Southall's favour and he was reinstated. The critics have not given up, however: they are still active and determined to reopen the inquiry.

What emerges from this episode, and seems to be confirmed from all the parental evidence in other sections of this book, is that doctors need to have open communication with parents; otherwise misunderstandings and resentment can follow. It is vitally important to involve parents in decisions about their very premature baby's treatment by making sure that they receive all relevant information so that they can make informed decisions. This means making sure that all parents, whatever their age, background or ethnic origin know exactly what the diagnosis and prognosis are likely to mean in the long term. Then the various measures and options available need to be made clear. The role of the neonatal nurse practitioner is important here: she can build lines of communication and support parents in putting their points of view over to Consultants. If there is trust between doctor and patient, the best interests of the baby is more likely to be served.

PART 5

The issue of justice and resources

Part 5 considers the care of very premature babies in the light of limited health care resources, and examines the hidden costs of caring for those that survive.

PART CONTENTS

14

The impact on society of saving very premature babies

> Where neonatal intensive care produces a child who will take its place in society, few would disagree that this is money well spent. It is when survivors require considerable help from the state in terms of special schooling or benefits, that doubts are raised about the cost effectiveness of neonatal units. As the NHS is increasingly expected to operate as a business, it can be anticipated that cost considerations will play a larger part in decisions about care.
>
> (Miller 1996, p. 137)

This statement emphasises the progressively difficult decisions that are emerging around the cost effectiveness of saving very premature babies. The dilemma of whether to continue expensive intensive neonatal care treatment can be exacerbated by infinite demands on finite resources. Cost effectiveness is now a priority in every area of the NHS agenda, as NHS reforms, political pressure and internal market philosophy make their mark. There is never enough money to meet all demands. Manpower, equipment and technology have become more expensive and along with new techniques have led to more choice and more demands. They have enabled practitioners to treat more illnesses than ever before, resulting in the increased possibility of keeping people alive for longer. Patient expectations have become more demanding and the rising proportion of elderly people in the population has added to expenses in other areas, such as social services. So economics and ethics interact more closely than ever and conflict arises between the value of human life and the social utility value of apportioning resources. Difficult decisions are unavoidable: priorities have to be set and there are bound to be winners and losers in the battle for resources.

According to Hadley (2000) it costs in the region of £800 per day to treat a premature baby who might be dependent on an intensive care unit for eighteen months; but of course, that is only the beginning of the story. The cost to society of servicing the needs of these children and their families will continue to the end of their lives, increasing as they get older. If we value their lives enough to save them at the beginning, is it not right and just that we should continue to value them as individuals throughout their lives and accord them the same rights and dignities that the rest of us expect?

This section looks at the principle of justice in relation to the allocation of health care resources, and some of the theories that can be applied to arguments justifying the fair distribution of resources. It will consider how the various theories might affect the distribution of priorities in the context of neonatal services, and how the justice and resource issue clearly affects the autonomy and equal opportunities of the disabled, particularly those people with profound and multiple learning disabilities. The legal guidelines that have evolved historically, and proposed legislation to uphold and protect their rights will also be considered.

THE PRINCIPLE OF JUSTICE

> Benefits and burdens within society should be apportioned in a way that is morally justifiable.
>
> (Sim 1997, p. 21)

Gillon (1985) reminds us that the Greek word for 'justice' is the same as their word for 'equality', i.e. equal shares for all. However, Aristotle rejected this notion and developed his own theory, saying that justice is a relative term: those who deserved more were owed more, and those who deserved less were owed less. 'Equal shares for all' only applied when those who deserved the same were given the same. In essence, Aristotle's principle of justice means that 'equals should be treated equally and unequals unequally in proportion to their relative inequalities' (Gillon 1985, p. 87). In other words, everyone should be treated equally, unless there are good reasons why some individuals deserve to be treated differently.

Earlier chapters have covered other moral principles, such as autonomy, beneficence and non-maleficence, which are applied within the doctor-patient relationship and apply to the treatment of the individual. The application of the principle of justice goes beyond the individual, as Singleton and McLaren (1995) indicate. In health care decisions, the idea that 'equals should be treated equally' applies in two areas: first, to decide what treatments should be made available within allocated resources, and second, to decide who should receive the treatments if there are not enough available for all those who need them.

Singleton and McLaren believe that a principle of justice needs to be designed to provide a just way of distributing benefits between individuals. Whilst the obligation to be fair to all people applies both to persons and governments, the rights of one individual become limited when they infringe on the rights of someone else.

As Gillon (1985) points out, the principle became widely accepted because it was non-specific. The relevant principles or inequalities are not laid down, and therefore it has been possible for both deontological and consequentialist theories of justice to emerge. Both have been found to have their limitations. Deontology can sometimes appear too inflexible: when duties or obligations have been found to conflict, difficulties have arisen about which should take precedence and about who decides which duties are relevant in the first place.

On the other hand, the consequentialist approach could be criticised for ignoring the rights of the individual, or for the fact that it is almost impossible to quantify the benefits and harms of actions in terms of health care.

Rawls' Theory of Justice

In his *Theory of Justice* (1973) Rawls attempted to incorporate both deontological and utilitarian approaches with respect for autonomy as its foundation. The theory stated that:

1. Everyone should enjoy maximum liberty (provided that liberty does not impinge on the liberty of others).
2. There should be equal distribution of resources unless an unequal division would be advantageous to the most disadvantaged in society. Rawls proposes that principles of justice should be decided from 'behind a veil of ignorance'. By this he meant that if those who met were from different walks of life in society and did not know what their role in society was to be, they would work out universal moral principles that would represent the fairest allocation of resources possible, to eliminate distribution on the basis of class or any other accidental circumstances, like, for instance, the ability to pay. Those who are most disadvantaged are benefited proportionally more, even though this may result in unequal distribution.

Justice can be roughly divided into two main areas: retributive justice and distributive justice. Retributive justice is involved with the administration of rewards and punishments, and is therefore mainly relevant to criminal law. It is with distributive justice that we shall be concerned in relation to the allocation of health care resources.

Distributive justice

According to Beauchamp and Childress (1989), distributive justice refers to the just distribution of services and goods in society structured by certain moral, legal and cultural rules and principles that are agreed implicitly and explicitly, under which individuals cooperate in society. Sim (1997) describes it as taking a comparative or non comparative form:

- Non comparative justice is where an individual receives what he/she needs and deserves.
- Comparative justice means that benefits received by one person are relative to those received by others.

Distributive justice in health care is dispensed on three levels.

Macro allocation

At this level, decisions are made about what proportion of national revenue should be allocated to health as opposed to other public services, like education, defence, transport, housing and social services. In his April 2002 budget speech Gordon Brown specifically targeted the National Health Service as the main area of funding. He promised that massive extra sums would be put into the Service, to compensate for the gross under-funding of previous governments. However, many economists queried whether the Health Secretary would actually receive all the funding he had been promised. It was pointed out that the Education Department would be staking their claims too. After all, Tony Blair came into office declaring that his government had three major priorities: education, education and education. Presumably the Secretary of State for Education will be reminding him of that when the allocation of resources is announced. Transport, too, is in major crisis and as Alan Watkins (2002) stated:

> In an age when a home visit by a doctor is as rare an event as a call from the Queen, the poor, the old and the vulnerable have to reach the surgery or health centres by public transport. Is this not as important as the treatment or advice they receive once they arrive there?
>
> (Watkins 2002, p. 23)

So we see the huge difficulties that arise when deciding who gets what at the macro allocation level. Every government department is competing to obtain the maximum possible from a finite pool of resources. Of course, some would say that the earmarking of funds by departments is almost an irrelevance, as treasury ministers ignore them anyway when they administer the finances.

Meso allocation

This is concerned with health care budgets, and what funds should be directed to which services (i.e. preventative medicine, research, different treatments, different hospitals). Decisions have to be made about whether scarce NHS budgets should be used to treat conditions that are not actually life-threatening (cosmetic surgery or infertility treatment, for example), whether funding should be allocated to treatments that can alleviate life-threatening conditions but which do not increase life expectancy, or whether funding should be put into treatments which can increase life expectancy, but are not likely to increase the quality of life. Neonatal intensive care units may well cause such dilemmas for policy makers.

In interviews with a few hospital administrators after the budget of 2002 it was interesting to see where they placed their priorities as far as their own hospitals were concerned. Some prioritised the purchase of new equipment, like operating theatres and surgical units. Others were more focused on increasing staffing levels and recruiting more doctors and nurses. The possibility of sustained investment and forward planning was another priority.

At the same time, members of the public who were interviewed and asked what improvements to the Health Service they would like to see, named the following list of priorities: better GP services, cutting hospital waiting times and lists, pay increases for doctors (and particularly for nurses), and better services for the old, the vulnerable and those who cannot speak for themselves.

Micro allocation

Here, decisions are made about what treatment patients will receive within the resources available at the time. Individual doctors decide which patients should be allocated life-saving treatment from their own departmental budgets: patients needing kidney dialysis or babies needing special care cots. Choices about who gets what at micro allocation level are dependent on what practitioners believe are the relevant features of patient care. How do they make such crucial decisions? What factors do they consider important when setting priorities about which patient receives which treatment? Are decisions influenced by the patient's age or family commitments, the needs of the patient, the chance of success of the treatment, or whether the illness is self-inflicted? Are decisions made on the basis of the doctor's view of the social usefulness or moral worth of an individual patient?

All these issues are important when ethical decisions regarding the just allocation of resources are made. Differing theories try to identify which characteristics enable one person or group to be entitled to more resources than another. However, it is important that however decisions are reached they can be defended impartially on solid ethical grounds, ruling out any arbitrary or biased judgement.

The theory of distributive justice attempts to establish a connection between the characteristics of persons and the morally correct distribution of burdens and benefits in society. As Sim (1997) puts it:

> Providing there are morally relevant differences between individuals, it is legitimate to provide them with different levels of therapeutic input. Therefore, to say that everybody has the right to health care, is not necessarily to say that everybody has a right to an equal *quantity* of health care.
>
> (Sim 1997, p. 116)

Downie and Calman (1987) agree that it is not wrong to discriminate in favour or against certain groups. Using Aristotle's model of 'treating like cases alike', they say that the key issue here is whether one can justify the decision in favour of one group over another in the context of scarce resources.

A concern for the principle of equity lies at the centre of NHS philosophy; it is putting the principle into practice that is the problem. For Heifetz (1996) equality of health care is neither possible nor necessary. Even though it would be physically and economically impossible to satisfy all demands, his emphasis lies with the principle of beneficence that, he says, entitles all citizens to have access to *good quality* health care. The NHS seems to place more importance on 'equal access' for 'equal need', which means that everyone should have an equal opportunity to use health service facilities whenever and wherever needed.

Of course, there are those, like Glover (1977), who would question whether such non-random measures could ever be adequately justified, since they give rise to questions about who decides, about how those decisions are reached, and about who is equal and who is unequal: if everyone has equal rights under the law, then everyone should have the right of access to all public services. Also there is the question of special groups in society (in which category we can place the very ill, very premature newborn). Should they be given access to special, expensive treatment with all its risks, over those less severely affected who have more chance of surviving undamaged? For Glover, the only really fair way to decide who to treat and where the resources should be spent is by random choice. However, for most practitioners and distributors of health care, this argument appears to be impractical, and as Appleby (1992) shows, there can be many interpretations of fairness:

- Equality of access to health care
- Equality of outcome of health care interventions
- Equal treatment of equal need.

However it is defined, Appleby identifies a consensus of feeling that equity in health care is important, and that patients want better and more successful treatment, noy only for themselves, but also for others.

Material principles of justice

Material principles of justice are those that identify the specific criteria used when decisions about fair distribution of resources are being weighed in the balance. Obviously, different interest groups will identify different criteria, which leads to disagreements about what material principles are valid. Beauchamp and Childress (1989) offer five alternatives to giving everyone an equal share:

1. To each person according to need
2. To each person according to effort
3. To each person according to free market exchanges
4. To each person according to contribution
5. To each person according to merit.

They point out that only one of the above might be acceptable to some, while others will embrace three or four, or even all of them. The important thing is that, whichever criteria are accepted, there must be a morally justifiable argument supporting the choice. Of course, one can see that dilemmas could arise when different material principles need to be applied in differing circumstances, because each of the five represents a *prima facie* obligation. Conflict seems inevitable when the competing moral claims are weighed against each other. However, the onus for establishing priorities lies with those in the government who make the decisions about which material principles to apply when allocating scarce resources, at both macro and meso level.

Looking at this model of justice, it certainly appears that in the case of the very ill premature baby, access to resources could only be justified by the first criterion; in no way could they, or any other child for that matter, qualify under any of the other four.

Medical triage

Heifetz (1996) introduces the concept of 'triage' for determining priorities in situations where difficult choices have to be made.

Triage is the term used for the sorting, sifting and selecting of priorities according to need, in order to produce the greatest benefit from limited resources. According to Heifetz this has two major components: allocation and rationing.

Allocation

This has to do with the decisions on a macro and meso level about how much money society decides to budget for health care. It is therefore mainly in the domain of government policy both at national and local levels. Ethical choices have to be made about where resources are targeted (health, education, housing and social services), weighing the benefits and harms to society as a whole. Decisions must be made about which sections of society will be favoured in a highly competitive market and which groups will lose out when the funding is allocated. Policy decisions are made about whether to spend money on, for example, popular and dramatic high technology which benefits a relatively small proportion of patients, or on the more mundane health education and preventative medicine which will reach far more of the population.

Rationing

Heifetz claims that equal access to the best medical help has never been available to all and therefore the rationing of health care is, and always has been, a fact of life. He points to the way doctors are forced to evaluate situations in intensive care, when they have to move one very ill patient out, so that another may take his place, even though, in other circumstances, the first patient would still be considered a candidate for ITU. With the triage system, the potential harm to each patient has to be balanced. This can inevitably lead to unpleasant and difficult choices at times; and new technological advances play a major factor in compounding the problem. Heifetz claims that eventually, if some sort of parameters are not drawn up, then the only criteria used will be:

1. First come first served
2. The potential quality of life
3. The social value of the individual to society.

The Quality Adjusted Life Year

It is hard to see now how the initial founding principles of the NHS can be delivered in today's economic climate. The belief that every life has equal value and that therefore everyone is entitled to equal treatment cannot always be taken for granted. Resources are scarce, so choices are unavoidable; a decision to use resources in one area inevitably means money cannot be spent in other areas.

One of the crucial factors in health care analysis is evaluation of the efficiency of the service, with the aim of producing a more effective and just distribution of resources. One of the ways of attempting this in recent years has been to introduce a cost/utility approach known as the QALY (Quality Adjusted Life Year). Medical intervention can usually be described as 'life enhancing' rather than 'life saving'; so in order to compare effects of different types or service or treatment there are two elements of health care to consider: 'quality of life' and 'length of life'.

According to Alan Williams (1985): 'The objective of economic appraisal is to ensure that as much benefit as possible is obtained from resources devoted to health care. In principle, the benefit is measured in terms of life expectancy adjusted for quality of life' (p. 76).

> The essence of a QALY is that it takes a year of healthy life expectancy to be worth 1, but regards a year of unhealthy life expectancy to be worth less than 1. The lower the value, the worse the quality of life of the unhealthy person (which is what the "quality adjusted" bit is about). If being dead is worth zero, it is in principle possible for a QALY to be negative. That is, for the quality of someone's life to be judged worse than being dead.
>
> (Williams 1985, p. 78)

So what is being proposed here is a utilitarian view that the best outcome possible can be defined in terms of the greatest number of QALYs produced. This can be used in decision-making at both macro and micro levels. At the macro allocation level, policy makers are concerned with maximising the cost/benefit; so treatments are assessed in relation the number of QALYs they would yield and their cost.

At the micro allocation level, selection of individual patients for treatments is assessed on how many QALYs treatment would yield for that person, against the cost per QALY. So it would be rational for decision makers to transfer resources away from very expensive treatments for the few, and towards less costly treatments to advantage more people in society. Singleton and McLaren (1995) argue that as decisions made at macro level must inevitably affect what happens at micro level, this system will automatically disadvantage a great many people, including some of the very damaged children who will survive to live lives of very poor quality.

More recently, other measures have been introduced to try and compensate the less able in society, namely the QWB (Quality of Wellbeing) and the DALY (Disability Adjusted Life Year). These are designed to take account of various levels of disability and their effect. Even so, according to Landman and Henley (1998), they only marginally affect results in favour of the severely disabled.

According to Sim (1997) a fair system of resource allocation needs certain safeguards built into it, which will protect the interests of those in society who are both vulnerable and powerless to speak out for themselves. He believes that a system that centres on maximising efficiency and effectiveness, by whichever means, will never achieve this. He prefers Rawl's concept that resources in society should be distributed in such a way that individuals who are the most disadvantaged should be assisted proportionately more, even though this might result in an unequal benefit to society generally speaking. In this way, Sim considers that the interests of justice are balanced against the desire for efficiency, but the needs of the individual are not entirely subordinated to the needs of the many.

IMPLICATIONS FOR NEONATAL CARE

> All individual clinical decisions about intensive care for the newborn need to be set in the context of shortage of resources and pressure on existing facilities.
>
> (Wyatt and Spencer 1992, p. 11)

Some would argue that the situation described earlier by Heifetz has already arrived in some areas of neonatal practice; Miller (1996) maintains that the shortage of special care cots is getting worse, especially in the south of England, and particularly in London. The problem is intensified by the shortage of qualified neonatal nurses. Salaries account for the largest proportion of the NHS budget, due to the high staff-patient ratio. Some hospitals are forced to refuse hundreds of requests for admissions from other hospitals because of a shortage of cots. Obviously, if alternative places were not found for those infants, there future would be very bleak.

Nevertheless, it is important to see the allocation of resources in the special care unit against the background of care for all infants. Treatment is often based on 'first come, first served' basis. In this situation, under the criterion of need, it is sometimes the case that larger, more mature babies may not be treated because smaller, immature infants, who are less likely to survive without damage, are taking up the space. Some would see it as wrong to allocate more money to expand the facilities for tinier babies, who may not survive intact, if it meant reducing beds for more mature infants, who have a good chance of a full and healthy life.

Summers (2002) says that nursing provision in special care units is consistently below recommended standards: one nurse for every three babies, compared to a ratio of one nurse to one patient in adult ITUs; and even that level is difficult to maintain, as recruiting specialist nurses is a problem owing to the stressful nature of the job. She quotes Professor Edwards from Queen Charlotte's Hospital, Hammersmith:

> Babies are not top of the Government's list of priorities. Babies don't vote.
> (Summers 2002, p. 37)

It seems that many who work in this field believe neonatal medicine to be the Cinderella service of the NHS and that national provision is at breaking point. Richard Cooke, Professor of Neonatal Medicine at Liverpool Women's Hospital goes on to add that the reason for more money being spent on heart surgery is because bankers keel over and demand resources, but babies don't say very much! (Summers, p. 37)

Although in global terms Britain is at the forefront of paediatric research, it is a sad reflection that much of the funding is raised by charities. According to Summers, 80% of incubators and ventilators are bought and paid for by charities, not by the NHS, and although the statistics say that 6% of the world is born preterm and 30% of people have heart disease, there is 33 times more research done into heart disease than into prematurity. The charity BLISS spent £120,000 pounds in 2001 buying ten new incubators for one leading neonatology unit in a London hospital because the existing ones were obsolete and could no longer be serviced. The same charity also funds training for neonatal nurses; the question is, should charities have to find money for basic equipment and training?

Nationally, there has been no specific planning regarding the care of very ill babies, until recently. However, government ministers are at present considering a major review which would mean a big reorganisation of both local and national care. The proposal is to develop a few specialist centres around the country, specially equipped with state of the art technology and highly trained staff, to deal with the growing number of very premature babies. Centres would be placed strategically, so that infants from local hospitals could be transferred for treatment, freeing up beds in general hospitals to treat the larger premature infants whose prognosis is better.

Miller (1996) makes the point that more very low birth weight babies are being born as a result of fertility treatment (which incidentally is usually administered in a private clinic), so multiple births are taking up cots in NHS maternity units, stretching resources to the limit. Twins are three times more likely to need intensive treatment than single babies; triplets are seven times more likely. So a situation can arise when the team may be treating triplets or quads belonging to one family, the result of which may be to deny another family the treatment for their only child. The estimated cost of these multiple births to the NHS is estimated at £60 million a year.

In response to this problem, a recent statement (reported by BBC News, 13th April 2002) by Ruth Deech, the former chairperson of the Human Fertilisation and Embryology Authority, suggested that new financial penalties should be introduced to curtail the number of multiple births as a result of IVF treatment. Fertility clinics were warned that they should consider paying towards the cost of multiple births to the NHS. It is estimated that the birth rate of triplets has more than doubled in the last fifteen years; the figure for the year 2000 rose to 285 and the hospital costs for the treatment of ten-week premature triplets amounts to £450,000.

As you would expect, doctors working in the private clinics which provide this service are critical of these proposals, arguing that there is only a small risk of multiple pregnancies and that most women need three or more eggs implanted in order for just one to survive. With the charge of anything up to £3000 for each attempt, it certainly seems that some women's chances of becoming pregnant would be greatly reduced if they had to return several times for treatment. One suggested solution to the problem has been for the introduction of compulsory insurance, taken out by IVF clinics to compensate the NHS should the situation arise; as has already been noted, there is no facility in private medicine for the care of very ill or very premature babies.

In 1984 a survey by Newns (Miller 1996) estimated the cost of a premature baby, whose birth weight was below 1000 grams and who survived treatment, to be £10,000. For those who did not survive, the cost was £1000. In today's terms, these figures are a gross underestimation, but even taking that into account, it would appear that in QALY terms, neonatal services are relatively cheap. However these figures do not reflect the full picture: they seem to assume that the survivors all escaped unscathed and do not take into account any future costs of services needed to support those who suffer severe impairment.

By contrast, in America an average hospital bill for the care of these tiny 'preemies' can amount to $100,000, plus the resources needed for lifelong ongoing care should they need it (Heifetz 1996).

Campbell and McHaffie (1995) argue that economics should not be a factor when considering quality of life issues, but do acknowledge that affordability of treatment or its consequences has to be a consideration. They feel that the quality of life issue should not involve judgements about a child's inherent value or social worth to the community in financial terms, but about their capacity for future health and wellbeing. Other factors should be considered, like their potential ability to reciprocate in human relationships and about the human cost to the child and family that will accrue if they survive into adulthood.

They advocate that these ethical issues should be policy led, and decided away from the clinical environment, while acknowledging that an infant who is deemed unable to develop those characteristics will inevitably take up resources which could be directed towards the support of other children who could form and sustain those kinds of relationships. In these kinds of circumstances Wyatt and Spencer (1992) advocate that there should be appropriate policies in place so that intensive care is withheld for babies under a certain gestational age and birth weight. In this way, no very premature baby falling below those criteria would block cots that may be needed for later infants born close to the limit of viability. In some cases decisions to begin treatment at the very outset can be difficult to reverse if things begin to get worse.

Certainly these issues need to be addressed honestly and realistically, and official parameters should be treated drawn up by paediatricians to determine which babies should and should not be treated. Those infants who do not match those conditions should be given palliative treatment only.

The Royal College of Paediatrics and Child Health (1997) also emphasises that treatment should not be governed by resources and should always be appropriate to the individual child. The document adopts a deontological stance and states that treatment should only be withheld or withdrawn in a 'no purpose' situation, when a child is expected to be so impaired (either physically or mentally) that life could be deemed an unbearable burden. Only then can it be ethically justified, because for the deontologist, the special obligations that a doctor has for the patient within a professional relationship override any general obligation to the wider community. Therefore, according to the Royal College, it is the duty of the doctor to prescribe appropriate treatment irrespective of any possible outcome.

However, they too have recognised that limitations on budgets do have implications for the use of expensive equipment as against spending the money elsewhere, for the benefit of more babies. They also make the point that medical teams working with these children and their families need to be highly skilled and trained, not only in clinical practice, but also in dealing with distressing, difficult and contentious issues. They strongly recommend that time, training and support are included in any ITU budget, so that high standards of care can always be maintained. Allocation of resources is never going to satisfy demands, and as new technologies develop, giving rise to more choices of treatment, doctors cannot avoid the fact that a decision about the management of one particular infant may have implications for the treatment of other, equally urgent, cases. The fact is, they do have other patients to consider, and conflicts of interest will be inevitable.

But what should the doctor do in these circumstances? Should he indicate to the patient (or parents, in the case of the neonate), that their wish for treatment has to be overridden in favour of his wider obligations to those whose needs are more urgent? Campbell and McHaffie (1995) claim that the doctor who argues that the Hippocratic Oath requires him/her to prescribe treatment for one particular patient, regardless of the needs of others, is being too idealistic and not admitting that decisions affecting allocation of resources are inescapable.

In contrast to the stance taken in the guidelines for the Royal College of Paediatrics and Child Health in this country, a survey in South Africa suggests that doctors and nurses in a neonatal special care setting, influenced by their awareness of economic constraints and the potential burden to families, exhibited strong utilitarian attitudes to resource allocation (Landman and Henley 1998).

Beauchamp and Childress (1989) point to possible dangers and tensions that could arise from adopting a too utilitarian approach; the doctor-patient relationship is based on trust. They write that during the early days of the NHS, doctors were trusted to deliver whatever treatment was deemed necessary, irrespective of cost. Patients and their families build up relationships with nurses and doctors, particularly in the area of neonatal care. Now, in the climate of scarce resources and NHS rationing, this relationship is in danger of being eroded because patients may be wary of treatments prescribed by doctors, in case decisions are made on the basis of cost and rationing of resources, rather than need.

Glover (1977) goes further, arguing that the process of 'interventionism' can threaten the society itself if some groups cannot feel confident that their interests are given equal weight with those of others. Decision-making about which groups should have preference over others means that, for Glover, the principle of equality is negated, because equality means that one person's (or group's) life is not more worthwhile than another. He questions how non-random choices are made: who makes the judgements, and how does the influence of pressure groups affect the final decision?

However, Glover does not rule out the possibility of weighing the potential quality of one life to be saved against another. The problem, as he sees it, is where the line of demarcation should be drawn about what is deemed 'a life worth living'. Miller's (1996) view, too, is that cost cannot be measured in economic terms only; although economic cost should never override the child's best interests, the cost to the whole family in relationship terms needs to be a strong consideration. As we have already seen, parental stress and siblings' feelings can be the cause of breakdowns in both health and partnerships, which in the end will inevitably affect the upbringing of a multiply disabled child.

Purcell (1997) argues that to take a purely deontological or utilitarian view is impossible when making real life decisions. Actions cannot be judged in terms of consequences or intentions alone. It is unlikely that a deontologist would take an action without also thinking of its consequences, just as a consequentialist would rarely act, thinking only of the outcome of his actions. As we have already seen, those practitioners who would like to take a purely deontological view on treatment are forced to admit that the principle of utility is an inescapable fact of life.

Questions of cost need to be considered not only in terms of material and economic costs to society, but also against other morally relevant factors such as the severity of the impairment, how effective the outcome is likely to be, and the emotional and social cost to parents and siblings.

However, weighing the cost against other morally relevant variables does not mean that, in general, no health care resources should be channelled towards individual high cost/high benefit treatment for smaller numbers of patients. In some cases, this may well be morally justified. Landman and Henley (1998) argue that there is a social conviction that the worse off individual has a greater moral claim to more health care than someone who is better off. So it seems reasonable to give weighted, rather than absolute, priority to the worse off in resource allocation and so mitigate the pitfalls of using too much for too few.

Robertson (1998) maintains that the arguments for non-treatment of babies with disabilities on the grounds that the social cost outweighs the benefit to the infant are flawed. He questions the idea that money potentially saved by withholding high cost intensive treatment for a few babies, would go to treat more babies who are more likely to survive undamaged. He argues that it does not necessarily follow that money saved in these areas would go to address the needs of other children. The funds may be swallowed up in other areas of health care that have nothing to do with neonatal resources. Therefore, because diagnoses about the future quality of life cannot be easily predicted, it would be unethical and, he believes, illegal, to sacrifice the lives of these babies on the grounds of social and economic cost.

IMPLICATIONS FOR THOSE CHILDREN WHO SURVIVE TO ADULTHOOD

Although the main emphasis of this book is saving those babies who have profound and multiple disabilities, many of the children who are saved and do grow to adulthood have varying degrees of disability. Much of the following material will have a bearing on all those very premature babies who survive, even those with less severe damage. Their numbers are growing, and all will need some sort of special help.

As we have noted, the impact of bringing up a child with severe or profound learning disabilities has a tremendous effect on family life, the cost of which is seen not only financially, but emotionally and socially too. One of the main facilities that these families rely on for support is the day centre, where the child or adult family member can go for outside stimulation and to widen their circle of friends. This amenity is not only beneficial to the person with learning disabilities, in that it offers the individual a degree of independence and autonomy, but it also gives parents or carers the chance to have time for themselves and to spend more quality time with the rest of the family or friends.

Some facts and figures

In a recent Mencap survey (ref: 162 MAYRE8/P) it was stated that

- In the UK around 200 children a week are born with a learning disability.
- Most families who have children with a learning disability get little or no emotional support after they are born.
- 20,000 adults with learning disabilities are living at home all day with their parents, with no day services or outside support.
- Four out of five children and adults with severe learning disabilities are not able to have even a short break away from home so that parents can take a rest from the stress of constantly caring for them.
- There are 60,000 day centre places available, costing £240 million per year.

According to a White Paper published by the Department of Health, 'Valuing People' (2001):

- There are around 1.2 million children and adults in England with a mild or moderate learning disability.
- There are approximately 210,000 people with severe or profound learning disabilities, about 120,000 of whom are adults of working age.
- 7% of adults with severe or profound learning disabilities are employed on a full-time basis. Those who are not employed, or are employed part-time, require access to other forms of day activity; for example, work experience, college courses or training of some sort.
- 80% of total budget costs for day services is taken up by day centres.
- There are 60,000 full-time equivalent day centre places. This does not cater for all the people who should be eligible for day services.
- According to government estimates, the shortfall in places amounts to around 20,000 full-time places for those with severe or profound learning disabilities. Others believe that the overall figure is nearer to 30,000, and that excludes people with less severe problems who also need some services due to health or other circumstances.

The legal framework

Over the past fifty years laws have been passed or changed to take account of society's growing awareness of the needs of the disabled. In 1953 The European Convention on Human Rights ratified The Treaty of Rome and in 1971 a Declaration on the Rights of Mentally Retarded Persons was passed at the United Nations General Assembly. Both were set up to protect human rights in general, and particularly those of people with disabilities, and stated that everyone has the right to 'life, liberty and security of person'.

The rules state that governments should ensure that disabled people are given equal opportunity in all areas of life: education, family, employment and medical care.

Under the Disability Discrimination Act 1995 anyone with a physical or mental impairment which has a substantial and long-term effect upon their ability to carry out normal day-to-day activities is deemed a disabled person. This description obviously encompasses a wide range of problems; as far as physical health is concerned it means 'the weakening or adverse change of a part of the body caused through illness, by accident or from birth' and includes sight and hearing impairment, cardiac and thoracic problems, paralysis of limbs and severe disfigurement. Mental damage includes all identifiable mental illnesses and learning disabilities.

Human rights campaigners now say that issues of discrimination against disabled people and breaches of their human rights are not being addressed, because the recommendations and rules enshrined in the UN Declaration lack authority: they are not legally binding and therefore not enforceable in England. Despite statements about equality and equal rights, prejudice is still prevalent in attitudes towards the disabled. Nevertheless, the Government has pledged to implement civil rights for people with disabilities. It set up a task force to investigate how best to put into operation wide-ranging and enforceable civil rights legislation. This initiative led to the Disability Rights Commission Bill 1999.

Some relevant Acts of Parliament passed in this country include the following:

- **1948 National Assistance Act – Section 29**. Local Authorities were given power to make arrangements for supporting those who were substantially and permanently 'handicapped'. Nowadays Local Authorities have a legal duty to provide day services, although they are not obliged to make them available for everyone with a learning disability (see 1990 NHS and Community Care Act below).
- **1970 Chronically Sick and Disabled Persons Act – Section 2**. This requires Local Authorities to arrange the provision of specific services, including transport to day services.
- **1977 National Health Services Act – Schedule 8 and Circular LAC (93) 10 Appendix 3**. This states that Local Authorities should provide day services for people with mental illness or learning disabilities.
- **1986 Disabled Persons (Services, Consultation and Representation) Act – Section 4**. This makes it a duty to assess the needs of a disabled person.
- **1986 Disabled Persons (Services, Consultation and Representation) Act – Sections 5 and 6**. These create a duty to assess the needs of disabled children leaving school or college.

- **1990 NHS and Community Care Act – Section 47**. This offers a structure for assessing the need for community care services. Local Authorities are duty bound to assess anyone who may be in need of community care and to make a decision about whether or not such services should be provided. Decisions are based on 'eligibility criteria' that the individual has to meet before being accepted for services. These criteria are based on the vulnerability of, and/or risk to the individual if they were not to receive the service. Crises in funding have meant the tightening up of eligibility criteria, so fewer people are meeting them and therefore less cash is spent.
- **1995 Disability Discrimination Act**. This made it illegal for any service provider to discriminate against disabled people. They are required to make 'reasonable adjustments' if disabled people find it impossible or unreasonably difficult to make use of their services. This includes shops, leisure facilities, churches, government and local council offices, hospitals, as well as places like solicitors' offices and courts. Service providers are also urged, in the Code of Practice, issued under the Act, to assess their facilities and ensure that they are 'user friendly' in favour of the disabled, and not wait until someone is forced to complain or point out the problems before they are addressed.
- **1999 Disability Rights Commission Act**. The Disability Rights Commission began operations in April 2000. It is an independent body set up by the Government to help achieve civil rights for disabled people. Its statutory duties are:
    1. To work to eliminate discrimination against disabled people
    2. To promote equal opportunities for disabled people
    3. To encourage good practice in the treatment of disabled people
    4. To advise the Government on the working of disability legislation.

To achieve these obligations, the Commission may help to arrange legal advice and services for any person with disabilities who needs to defend their civil rights; or they may provide an independent conciliation service in disputes between service providers and disabled people. Another role is to determine how successful the law is in achieving equal rights for the disabled.

The Commission also acts as an information service, providing and advising on codes of practice to anyone who needs guidance on their statutory duties with regard to disabled people; this may include employers, service providers or disabled people themselves. They also monitor and investigate the treatment of disabled people and will carry out formal enquiries within specific organisations, if there is any complaint about discriminatory action.

What resources and day provision is offered at present?

Mencap recently published a report entitled 'A life in the day', in response to the Government White Paper. In it, they draw attention to the problems that Local Authorities face when attempting to fund day services for people with special needs. Financial constraints due to cuts in budgets have resulted in many Authorities being forced to reduce these facilities; some are barely managing to provide even the minimum to satisfy statutory requirements. In some cases this has meant the complete closure of day centres, in others there has been a reduction in the number of days or hours per week offered to individual service users. This has particularly affected people who are living in residential settings; the rationale seems to be that their needs are already being catered for, therefore there is no need for additional day centre provision.

As Mencap point out, these assumptions are flawed on several counts: some people moved into residential homes on the understanding that day care would be provided on a certain number of days in the week; people are not being reassessed before their services are cut; day centres have a different function from care homes. They enable individuals to experience a wider range of activities and friendship groups, for which residential care homes are neither equipped nor staffed; nor are they provided with the funding or the expertise to undertake the added responsibility.

There also appears to be evidence that eligibility criteria are being tightened, which means that many more people with mild or moderate learning disabilities are being completely refused day care. Another allegation is that some Authorities are closing day centres before any other practical alternatives are in place and are offering cheaper and inferior services in their place: activities such as group outings and sending people on college courses that have no real purpose or aim.

Another problem arising from cost-cutting budgets has been the introduction of charges for day centre attendance and transport. Although no figures are available, and Authorities are not required to publish the information, it is nevertheless suspected that many people are barred from using the facilities because they cannot afford the fares or entry fee. According to the Mencap report, people with learning disabilities and their families are becoming increasingly alarmed and angered by this development, especially when there appears to be little or no consultation and when they believe it is to help address a budget deficit within social services.

Transport costs do amount to a substantial part of the day services budget, particularly for rural areas, when they can add up to one quarter of all existing resources. The high cost is due to the very long journey that some people have to make in order to attend a day centre. Sometimes, people can be on the bus for hours at a time each way, making it both tiring and time consuming. High costs of transport and lengthy journey times have been major factors in decisions to provide more community-based facilities. However, paradoxically, people still often have to meet at the original day centre before moving to other activities; they travel to the day centre as before, only to make the journey back again to participate in some other activity within their home community!

The particular problems associated with people with profound and multiple learning disabilities

The problems associated with resource issues and justice are multiplied and magnified when it comes to servicing the needs of people with profound and multiple learning disabilities. In their report, Mencap emphasise this fact and point out a number of issues that are particular to this group of disabled people. One of the main dilemmas is that of segregation. Some never receive any kind of day services at all; parents are left to care for them all day, every day, because such specialised services are not available in their area. The impact on the lives of those families is devastating.

Those who do receive day care are catered for in special units run by social services, or provided by the NHS, which means that they suffer a double segregation: they are missing not only the stimulation from the wider community, but also the company of other service users with more moderate learning disabilities. The range and quality of the activities offered are often unsuitable because resources are scarce and mainly directed towards those with less severe disabilities. As we have already seen, in recent years there has been a change in expectations for the profoundly and multiply disabled child, particularly in the field of education. Multisensory programmes of work and intensive communication techniques encourage more interaction; choices are offered about what kind of food they would like or what type of activity they prefer.

Staffing levels are also a problem. Turnover is high in these centres for many reasons: lack of training facilities can make caring for people with profound and multiple learning disabilities a frustrating occupation, as lack of feedback and failures in communication make life very difficult. All in all, the particular needs of people with profound and multiple learning problems are not being met; therefore their access to equal opportunities is being denied. Obviously, some activities are not practical or feasible, and those that are can be very costly because of the high ratio of staff to client: it is usually a one-to-one situation. Other activities are both enjoyable and beneficial: hydrotherapy pools and multisensory environments can be wonderfully relaxing and therapeutic places. If they were situated in leisure centres they could be open for everyone to enjoy and the problems of segregation would be solved. Unfortunately, at the moment they can only be found in specialist centres which the general public do not usually frequent. As the Mencap report emphasises:

> Great care should be taken to ensure that these resources do not become the be all and end all of day services for people with profound and multiple learning disabilities. There is no reason why people with such disabilities should not be enjoying real activities in the community and building their own circle of friends like any other person. It is only economics and convenience that dictate that people with profound and multiple learning disabilities should spend their days together. Day services should instead be driven by a person's choice and potential.
>
> (Mencap 'A Life in the Day', p. 31)

There are many community-based activities in which people with profound and multiple learning disabilities can participate if they can receive the right support. I know that a favourite pastime for the children I taught was a visit to a garden centre, smelling the flowers and touching the different textured plants and trees.

They also enjoyed stopping off for a coffee or glass of lemonade and cake in the cafeteria. Nearly all of them needed help with feeding, which takes time and patience, if they have problems chewing or swallowing. If these activities are to be as trouble-free as possible it means the provision of special toilet facilities in public places; disabled toilets are not adequate when an adult with profound and multiple learning disabilities needs to be toileted and changed. In this situation, adult-sized changing tables are a necessity. Unfortunately, these facilities are few and far between: they are expensive to install and service providers are either unwilling or cannot afford to provide them. The result is that in planning community-based activities for the multiply disabled, the type of amenities available always restricts teachers and carers. Almost without exception, these people are wheelchair bound, and most will have their own personally designed seating, to suit their particular disability, from which they cannot be removed. They will always need special transport, that is, a vehicle with a tail lift, before they are able to participate in any outside activities. It is a problem that can be overlooked: these vehicles are not cheap, but adequate resourcing is vital if the multiply disabled are to have access to amenities within the community.

In the end, the quality of services for children and adults with profound and multiple learning disabilities is reliant on how Government and individual Local Authorities define their priorities. The problem for the planners is that there are increasing numbers of people within this group, as more and more severely disabled children survive to adulthood.

So where do we go from here?

The latest government proposals for changes in day services for people with a learning disability were initiated in March 2001, in a White Paper entitled 'Valuing People: A new strategy for learning disability for the 21st century'. In this document it is proposed that the traditional role of day centres for people with learning disabilities run by Local Authorities be reappraised and modernised, so that resources become more flexible and geared to the needs of individuals and their active involvement in developing skills and potential. The report appears to recognise that people with severe and profound learning disabilities have the right of access to local amenities that will enhance their lifestyle and give them as much autonomy as possible. Actually delivering the goods may be another story, which I discovered when visiting a club for the disabled run entirely by parents and volunteers, on church premises, in May 2002.

The group consisted of about 25 young men and women with moderate or severe learning disabilities; three or four had profound and multiple learning disabilities. There were about five helpers, all either parents or siblings of the club members. The club meets every week for two hours, between 7.00 and 9.00pm. Activities ranged from table tennis, indoor football, table games and craft work. The organiser, herself a parent of one of the youngsters, told me that all but two of the young people lived at home. She maintained that only two of the group had any day care and that none had any sort of employment or further education; this was the only activity provided for these people; and it was run by volunteers on church premises. There was no social services or Local Authority input. She confirmed that more stringent criteria are being used when assessing people for places in day centres: nearly every member of this group had been denied access.

One young man of about 30 years of age was caring for his 60+-year-old mother, who had recently had a mastectomy; the carer finding herself in the position of being cared for by her disabled son. Another man of 40 years had been in residential accommodation, but when it was closed down he was sent back to live with his ageing father who was over 80 years old and finding it impossible to cope.

The thing that struck me about the encounter was the lack of militancy among those volunteers; the attitude was one of resignation that this is how it had always been and things have not changed. They seemed to have little faith in anything happening to improve things in the near future.

This is just one small unit in a northern town. I wonder how many others there are, in the same situation, up and down the country?

Mencap have outlined some principles which they believe could act as guidelines for a modernised service. They approve of the proposed movement from large traditional centres and recommend smaller community-based services that enable people with learning disabilities to develop as individuals, participating in decisions and making choices about their lives.

Of course, in order to achieve these goals and make the service more effective, more expertise is required to pinpoint the specific needs of people with severe or profound learning disabilities. Planning and integration of resources and budgeting, between other agencies and local service providers, could bring about a fundamental change in the accessibility and quality of service.

What kind of services do we need?

The following is an outline of some of the key principles and recommendations made in the excellent Mencap document 'A life in the day', that are based on the idea that people with learning disabilities, whether moderate, severe or profound, should enjoy equal rights and opportunities in today's society.

> Mencap is calling on local authorities and social services departments in particular, to rise to the challenges contained in Valuing People and to take this opportunity to develop day services which meet the dreams and aspirations of people with learning disability.
>
> (David Congdon, Mencap Director of Public Affairs)

Recommendations for the Government

To issue guidelines to Social Service Departments on the modernisation of day services and to provide them with enough funding to enable them to make good quality day services available for all those who need them.

Recommendations for Social Services

- That services are founded on person-centred planning; looking at individuals' needs and choices and making sure that activities have real purpose and are community based.
- That all service users get the correct level of service, at the time they choose; even when this may mean weekend or evening provision.
- To work with other agencies including voluntary groups and employers, to provide flexible and wide-ranging amenities and resources, within the local community.
- To cater for the specific needs of people with profound and multiple learning disabilities.

• To work with the new Connexions agency to ensure school leavers are provided with appropriate education, employment, training and day services.
• To assess and take account of the needs of carers by establishing advisory groups consisting of people with learning disabilities and their carers.
• That good quality staff training is available and that staff are supported in their roles.

Of course, all these recommendations cannot be achieved by goodwill alone. Extra money will be needed and it is here that Mencap introduces a cautionary word, for the Government White Paper says little about providing a flexible or full-time service, or locally-based resource centres. Another concern is that there is no clear indication of how much money will be available or when it will be released. The fear is that existing day centres will close before any alternatives have been set up, which will be disastrous for the people who use the services and their families. Other competing priorities could mean that the money that is earmarked for the modernisation is less than anticipated; funding expected from the Learning Disability Development Fund is dependent upon money that cannot be released until long-stay hospitals have been closed. Then there will be other departments laying claim to some of the cash. The Learning Development Fund budget for 2002-03 was £42 million, which has to be divided between a number of priorities, including day services. This figure is nowhere near enough to put the proposals into practice; this would cost at least another £140 million per year, if the 20,000 people without services at present were to be provided for.

So while 'Valuing People' sets out noble objectives, it does not commit the Government to any increase in services for people with learning disabilities. Mencap sums it up:

> Mencap fully supports the modernisation of day services. It wants to see new and innovative services for people with a learning disability that will enable them to develop and control their own lives. Mencap does not doubt the Government's commitment to the principles contained in Valuing People, but we fear that unless more funding is provided, this vision will not be achieved.

Local Authorities are required to have their initial plans for the modernisation process in place by January 2003, and full implementation is to take place by 2006.

CONCLUSION

In terms of the care and resource allocation for babies who survive with profound and multiple disabilities, Rawls' approach would give weight to the argument that because as they get older, they will represent one of the most disadvantaged groups in society, both socially and economically, they should also be the recipients of the greatest benefits. At the micro allocation level, this should have a 'trickle down' effect: in every hospital the neonatal intensive care unit would be fully equipped with better staffing levels and more cots and equipment, so that every baby could be treated according to its particular need in every hospital.

In terms of macro allocation this would mean a greater injection of cash into health, social services and education budgets, so that all those resources needed by the growing child and its family could be better met. From the viewpoint of the deontologist, this would help redress the balance imposed by their disabilities and help them gain maximum liberty and autonomy, despite their relative inequalities.

The problem for the Government is that the more efficient we become at saving babies initially, the more will survive with some sort of disability; this inevitably will lead to a higher cost for society as a whole in terms of providing all those resources. We must ask questions about whether the services provided for those who survive, impair or enhance their quality of life; and whether in fact considerations about future care are taken into account when decisions about withdrawing or withholding treatment are made. For, if the sophisticated technology is made available for saving lives, there is an implicit moral obligation on the part of society that adequate services will be provided for those who survive with severe disabilities and their families. Questions need to be addressed, not only about how priorities are decided, but about what information is available to those who are responsible for resource allocation at local government level. For, as Mittler (1988) points out, there are still many disabled adults who are living close to or below the official poverty line, and while many of the younger generation enjoy a better quality of life in the community, others (mainly older people) are still living in poor conditions, with minimal treatment and staffing.

The problem lies in society itself, according to Wyatt and Spencer (1992). Despite the laws that have been passed to provide better facilities for the disabled it is because of society's ambiguity towards them that resources are patchy and under-funded. In my own experience, taking a profoundly disabled youngster into the community can pose great problems for some of the general public. There are those who feel a genuine compassion and want to help; there are those who feel compassion, but do not know how to react, so they try not to notice; and there are those who are openly hostile. Some of the latter have not bothered to conceal their disapproval, even disgust sometimes.

Mittler (1988) argues that while most people accept the idea of community care in theory, in reality arguments are often put forward to counter the transfer of resources to these amenities. Cuts in public expenditure often mean the erosion of the principle that underpins provision of full access to community services for the disabled. Mittler cites a former government minister as saying that if the disabled want to be seen as citizens in the mainstream of society, they too must face up to the harsh realities and accept their share of hardships just like other people. As Mittler rightly indicates:

> No question here of positive discrimination, no allowance for the low base rate from which they were starting, little recognition of the principle of special need.
>
> (Mittler 1988, p. 155)

Certainly, the very close relationship between moral, clinical and economic factors in decision-making is inescapable. Therefore the need to establish priorities is essential.

One of the criticisms aimed at the role and use of QALYs, QWB and DALY at a macro allocation level is their emphasis on maximising cost/benefit, sometimes to the detriment of equality of basic opportunities (Landman and Henley 1998). For the decision makers concerned with the treatment of very premature babies there are a number of tensions that underline the difficulties of balancing the principle of equality with the idea of maximising overall welfare. On the one hand, equality requires that individual children have equal access to all those conditions necessary for their future development; on the other hand, given the scarcity of resources, it is rational to strive for the most beneficial outcome for the majority of babies.

Setting priorities based solely or predominantly on Aristotle's principle of equality could mean employing huge resources in treating the most disabled, so giving them the chance to develop to their full potential, but taking the risk of pouring money into a 'bottomless pit'. On the other hand, setting priorities based largely on maximising general wellbeing may mean that certain children will have to be abandoned. As Mittler (1988) points out, anyone who is familiar with the services currently available for disabled people will know how unevenly distributed they are. Some authorities provide excellent facilities, while others struggle with under-staffing and under-funding.

Legislation and philosophical debate both endorse the view that people with mental and physical disabilities are valued citizens in society, with equal rights and responsibilities to anyone else. In theory, this means that they are given the same opportunities to exercise their autonomy as any able-bodied person; making as many choices about their lives as they are able. This has been particularly important for mentally disabled individuals, for in the past most people with severe learning disabilities were considered incapable of making any rational choices. Even the most commonplace choices, that most people take for granted, like what to wear or what to eat, were taken out of their hands. As Mencap comments:

> Services should offer the opportunity for people to decide what they want to do, explore their potential and gain independence.

I remember a vivid example of the way one young girl's life was changed by giving her the chance to choose her own clothes. Judith was a very pretty seventeen-year-old pupil; she had no physical disability, but was very severely mentally disabled, resulting in sudden eruptions of violent behaviour towards anyone who happened to be near her. Consequently, taking her shopping could become nightmarish, as we never knew whether she would be able to control herself in a crowded place. As a result, her carers usually bought her clothes for her. This was not always successful: if she did not like what they had bought, she simply refused to cooperate in dressing herself, and would sometimes take off the offending garments in public, much to the embarrassment of teachers, carers or perfect strangers if they happened to be around.

This became a real problem, until her carer hit on the idea of trying to persuade some of the high street shops to cooperate by allowing her to take a range of different outfits back to the house where they lived in the community, so that Judith could choose the ones she preferred. To their credit a few of the chain stores in town listened to the story and agreed to a trial period.

This simple act changed Judith's life and was a revelation to everyone else. We discovered that Judith had a real eye for fashion and colour. She was very clear about what she liked and disliked and was able to mix and match outfits with the flair of a professional. The other interesting feature of the enterprise was that she seemed to be able to match the colour of her clothes to her mood that morning: if she arrived dressed in bright red we knew to watch out, we were in for trouble!

This simple decision cost nothing financially, only the cooperation of local businesses.

Unfortunately, even though in theory society seems to be in favour of equality of rights and privileges for the disabled, in practical terms it is not always the case. The declarations enshrined within legislation are vague and open to varied interpretations. Phrases like 'subject to the availability of resources' or 'to the maximum extent possible' can be used to deny opportunities in education, leisure activities and social services. One mother illustrates this point in a letter to The Guardian newspaper; she describes how her Local Authority has cut the funding to three resource centres that service the area in which she lives. The result is that her mentally disabled 10-year-old is being deprived of the opportunity to develop independence and experience life outside his family. She made the point that because of his disabilities, he rarely gets invited to friends for tea or parties, and certainly never has the opportunity of a 'sleepover' like any other normal youngster. The cutbacks in facilities have curtailed almost all of his chances for socialising with anyone outside his family and school. She ends her letter with the words:

> I don't intend to take these cuts lying down. I will find more energy from somewhere. It's amazing what a motivator a fight for your child is. I will get a life for him.
>
> (Claire McCarthy, Guardian Society 24th April 2002)

Action groups comprising of parents and the disabled themselves are now making their voices heard, demanding that they are given access to the same quality of services as other members of society. In recent years, we have seen scenes of dissent from people in wheelchairs with placards outside the gates of Downing Street, protesting about disability issues; one or two individuals going as far as causing disturbances and resisting arrest.

In introducing his budget of April 2002, Gordon Brown increased National Insurance contributions by 1%. In doing so, he acknowledged that it would not be a popular decision, but said that it would define the character of the country and test our commitment and resolve. For years now, opinion polls have been reporting that people are willing to make sacrifices and contribute more in taxation to improve public services; it will be interesting to see how these extra resources are distributed and whether those in the greatest need will be in receipt of the benefits to which they are entitled. The immediate reaction, from most people, was that the increases were both necessary and worthwhile: we were hoping for better facilities, particularly for those members of society who are vulnerable and cannot speak for themselves.

15

Conclusion

In my Introduction I explained my reasons for writing this book. I was perplexed: on the one hand, knowing and working with profoundly impaired children has helped me to appreciate their individual qualities as human beings; yet I wondered whether, in the light of the immense problems encountered by these children and their families, plus the great burden on medical, educational and social resources, it would have been better if they had not been saved by intensive treatment in the first place. My main concerns were to do with sanctity and value of life issues, personhood and the just allocation of scarce resources.

I am now satisfied that the sanctity of life doctrine is very difficult to sustain separately from quality of life considerations. Neither the courts nor the theologians can sustain a doctrine that says that *every* life has intrinsic value and therefore should be saved at all costs. It follows that some lives are more valuable than others, and I think this reality needs to be addressed when policies are being formulated for intensive neonatal care.

In fact, it seems that selective treatment of the newborn is already well established in hospitals all over the country. Doctors are forced into making choices daily about which child should live and which should be left untreated. Therefore I agree with those who say that there should be a much more open and honest debate about the issues.

The child who is suffering irreversible brain damage will in the future be totally dependent on others. They will be at the centre of the family's life for as long as they live. The future quality of life for the baby will be reliant mainly on the quality of life enjoyed by the whole family; the two are completely interrelated and so need to be weighed together. Of course, it is true that many families cope remarkably well, and even turn a devastating situation into something positive and meaningful; but it is also true that for many more, caring for the growing child often creates parental and sibling stress, leading to family breakdown. The fact that society has changed and that family life is changing is another factor to be considered when thinking about the future of these very damaged infants. For single parents and divorced couples the problems only multiply.

In the light of this I see the notion of 'substituted judgement' as very helpful; for if this very premature baby is a person they should be granted the dignity and respect given to any other person in the same situation. Therefore one should try and ascertain what choices the child would make if it were aware of its present state of disability and could take all the factors surrounding the family situation into consideration. Whatever the outcome, it can be assumed that the decision will be one which is in the best interests of the child.

Another matter that is of obvious importance is that of the relationship between doctor and parents. All the guidelines and articles on the subject emphasise the value of close liaison between the neonatologist and parents during treatment. However, it does seem that while many doctors do try to comply, and show a deep compassion for the babies and their families, there are still some who persist in paternalistic attitudes and approaches to the care of the child. Parental autonomy is often undermined, sometimes unwittingly no doubt, and parents are kept in the dark about the severity of their child's condition. Nevertheless it is undoubtedly true that most parents wish to be told the truth about diagnosis and prognosis and doctors have a moral obligation to pass on such information. Having said that, I recognise that it is not always possible to be absolutely accurate in assessing any damage; but we are told that with new levels of sophistication in technology things are improving all the time.

The Royal College of Paediatrics and Child Health have gone a long way in guiding medical practitioners on what can be deemed correct practice within the legal limits; but I feel that even they have not really addressed the very complicated problem of how scarce resources inevitably impinge on decision making in the clinical situation. Just allocation of these resources causes great dilemmas now; but I am positive that in the future the problem will become a great deal worse in neonatal units, if babies are saved at earlier and earlier gestational ages.

We really do need to examine carefully the way we order

priorities. I strongly believe that if we as a society subscribe to the technology that can save these tiny infants, then we also have a moral obligation to make sure that resources are in place to support them and their families as they grow to adulthood. That of course implies that there has to be the political will to tackle the massive increases in finance which will be needed in the future. Gordon Brown has made a start with the increase to the NHS budget. Whether any of the extra funds will find their way into neonatal care is up to others. The problem will not go away, and unless we address these vital concerns, the number of very premature babies who survive with profound mental and physical disabilities will keep on increasing and they, their families and society will pay the escalating price.

I began the book with the example of one very premature infant who had survived unscathed to lead a healthy and happy life. I would like to finish on another positive note. Just as I was coming to the end of my writing, the following report, by Charles Begley, was printed in The Independent on Sunday on May 26th 2002.

World's tiniest baby goes home healthy

Against all odds the world's tiniest baby is recovering at home with her mother this weekend after astounding doctors in Italy with her fight for survival. The baby, nicknamed Pearl by the medical team at Florence's Careggi Hospital, was so small she could fit snugly into the palm of your hand. Although her birth weight of 285gm is around an ounce heavier than the Guinness Book of Records' smallest, Pearl's weight plummeted to 255gm shortly afterwards. This makes her the tiniest human being ever to survive. Dr Firmino Rubatelli hailed her survival as a "true and proper miracle" and said he was confident she would go on to lead a normal life.

That is indeed a wonderful outcome, from what must have been a very traumatic three months for both baby and parents. We applaud the doctors, nurses and all those who had some part in her recovery, for all the effort, skill, technology and resources whose use has been vindicated by such a worthwhile outcome. From the newspaper report it appears that Dr Rubatelli has given her parents every hope that her tenuous start will not mar her future chances in life.

Appendix

SERVICES AND HELPLINES AVAILABLE TO PARENTS

BLISS: The premature baby charity
Telephone: 0500 618140 (Freecall)
Website: www.bliss.org.uk
This charity gives advice and provides resource information about premature babies.

Cerebra 2002: A foundation for the brain injured infant
Telephone: 0800 328 1159 (Freephone)
Website: www.cerebra.org.uk
A free information service offering support to parents of brain injured children. Gives information on a range of topics: education, toys for special needs, a library service, therapies available. Can also put parents in touch with each other so that support and information can be shared. The organisation also commissions and funds research into cerebral palsy.

Child Death Helpline
Telephone: 0800 282 986 (Freephone)
Website: www.childdeathhelpline.org.uk
An organisation of professionals and parents working in partnership to provide a listening service and support for parents, siblings, grandparents and anyone else who has been affected by the death of a child of any age. It is based at Great Ormond Street Hospital, staffed by volunteers and supported by a professional team. It is not a counselling service.

MENCAP
Telephone: 020 7454 0454
Website: www.mencap.org.uk
This is a leading UK charity working with people with a learning disability and their families and carers. Its work includes supporting families, with advice and practical help, befriending people with a learning disability who are cut off from the community, and helping people with profound disabilities to learn to communicate. The organisation aims to help people with a learning disability to enjoy their lives through social and leisure activities, and to teach people with a learning disability the everyday skills they need to be independent.

SANDS (Stillbirth and Neonatal Death Society)
Telephone: 020 74365881
This Helpline is open between 10am and 3pm Monday to Friday.
There is an answerphone available at other times.
Office Number: 020 7436 7940
Fax: 02074363715
Email: support@uk-sands.org
SANDS is a national self-help organisation which has charitable status. It is run by volunteers whose purpose is to befriend and support bereaved parents and families who have suffered a stillbirth or neonatal death.

Tommy's: The Baby Charity
Telephone: 020 7620 0188
This number is staffed between 9am and 5.30pm Monday to Friday.
Fax: 020 7928 6628
Email: mailbox@tommy's.org
Tommy's is a charity that funds research, and offers education and information to anyone wishing to understand and prevent premature birth, miscarriage and stillbirth.

References

Allen M C, Donohue P K, Dusman A E 1993 The limit of viability: neonatal outcome of infants born at 22-25 weeks' gestation. New England Journal of Medicine 329 (22): 1597-1601

Angelini D J, Knapp C N F, Hankins L C et al (eds) 1986 Obstetrics. Prentice Hall, Pearson Education, Harlow

Appleby J 1992 Financing health care in the 1990s. Open University Press: Buckingham

Atkinson, Crawforth 1995 All in the family: siblings and disability. In: Action for Children. National Children's Home Publications, London

Beauchamp T L, Childress J F 1989 Principles of biomedical ethics 3rd edn. Oxford University Press, Oxford

Begley C 2002 World's tiniest baby goes home healthy. Independent on Sunday 26th May: 11

Beresford B 1995 Times they are a-changin'. Community Care 1099: 20

Boseley S 2001 Renegade or genius? The Guardian [G2] 16th Oct

Braine D, Lesser H (eds) 1988 Ethics, technology and medicine. Avebury Press, Aldershot

Brazier M 1992 Medicine, patients and the law. Penguin, London

Brechin A, Walmsley J (eds) 1989 Making connections. Hodder and Stoughton, London

Brindle D, Roseley S 1997 Parent's telling point on disability. The Guardian 27th Mar: 11

Byrne E, Cunningham C, Sloper P 1988 Families and their children with Down's Syndrome. Routledge and Kegan Paul, London

Campbell A G, McHaffie H E 1995 Prolonging life and allowing death: infants. Journal of Medical Ethics 21 (6): 339-344

Campbell A, Gillett G, Jones G 2001 Medical ethics. Oxford University Press, Oxford

Campbell N 1999 When care cannot cure: medical problems in seriously ill babies. In: Kuhse H, Singer P Bioethics: an anthology. Blackwell, Oxford

Collins V 1968 Limits of medical responsibility in prolonging life. Guides to decisions. Journal of the American Medical Association 206 (2): 389-392

Cooke K, Bradshaw J, Lawton D et al 1986 Child disablement, family dissolution and reconstitution. Developmental Medicine and Child Neurology 28 (5): 610-616

Cunningham C, Davis H 1985 Working with parents. Open University Press, Buckingham

Davies D K 1999 Ethics in the neonatal intensive care unit. http://www.preemie-l.org/ethicsdd.html accessed 03/09/01

Davis N 1993 A contemporary deontology. In: Singer P A companion to ethics. Blackwell, Oxford

Department of Health 2001 Valuing people: a new strategy for learning disability for the 21st century. HMSO, London

Downie R S, Calman K C 1987 Healthy respect. Faber and Faber, London
Draper H 1996 Consent in childbirth. In: Frith L Ethics and midwifery. Butterworth-Heinemann, Oxford
Dworkin R 1993 Life's dominion. Harper Collins, London
Edwards S 1997 The moral status of intellectually disabled individuals. Journal of Medicine and Philosophy 22 (1): 29-42
Englehardt H T Jr 1975 Ethical issues in aiding the death of young children. In: Kohl M Beneficent euthanasia. Prometheus Books, New York
Ethics Advisory Committee 1997 Withholding and withdrawing life saving treatment in children: a framework for practice. Royal College of Paediatrics and Child Health, London
Fairburn G, Fairburn S (eds) 1988 Ethical issues in caring. Avebury Press, Aldershot
Featherstone H 1980 A difference in the family. Basic Books, New York
Ferguson P R 1997 Causing death or allowing to die? Developments in the law. Journal of Medical Ethics 23 (6): 368-372
Ferngren G B 1987 The images dei and the sanctity of life. In: McMillan R C Euthanasia and the newborn. Kluwer, Dordrecht
Fetus & Newborn Committee, Canadian Paediatric Society & Maternal-Fetal Medicine Committee, Society of Obstetricians & Gynaecologists of Canada 1994 Management of the woman with threatened birth of an infant of extremely low gestational age. Canadian Medical Association Journal 151: 547-553
Finnis J 1999 Abortion and health care ethics. In: Kuhse P, Singer P Bioethics: an anthology. Blackwell, Oxford
Fletcher J 1998 The cognitive criterion of personhood. In: Pence G E Classic works in medical ethics. McGraw Hill, Boston MA
Forshaw S 1995 Treatment without consent. Nursing Times 91 (1): 27-29
Frader J E, Watchko J 1997 Futility issues in paediatrics. In: Zucker M B, Zucker H D Medical futility. Cambridge University Press, Cambridge
Frith L (ed) 1996 Ethics and midwifery. Butterworth-Heinemann, Oxford
Gallagher J J, Vietze P M (eds) 1986 Families of handicapped persons. Brookes, Baltimore MD
Gillon R 1985 Philosophical medical ethics. Wiley and Son, Chichester
Glover J 1977 Causing death and saving lives. Penguin, London
Goodall J 1986 The chimpanzees of Gombe. Harvard University Press, Cambridge MA
Hack M, Wilson-Costello D, Friedman H et al 2000 Neurodevelopment and predictors of outcomes of children with birth weights of less than 1000 grams. Archives of Paediatric Medicine 154 (7): 725-731
Hadley C 2000 Life in the balance. The Independent Magazine 12th Nov: 39-42
Harris J 1985 The value of life. Routledge, London
Harrison H 2002 Preemie Personality - Dr Mary Shirley (1939) http://www.comeunity.com/premature/research/helen/-1939.html accessed 17.01.02
Hayry M 1998 Ethics committees, principles and consequences. Journal of Medical Ethics 24 (2): 81-85
Heifetz M D 1996 Ethics in medicine. Prometheus Books, New York
Hostler J 1988 The sanctity of life and the sanctity of death. In: Braine D, Lesser H Ethics, technology and medicine. Avebury Press, Aldershot
Hursthouse R 1987 Beginning lives. Blackwell, Oxford
Jackson J 2001 Truth, trust and medicine. Routledge, London
Kennedy I, Grubb A 1995 Medical law. Butterworth, London
Keown D 1995 Killing, karma and caring: euthanasia in Buddhism and Christianity. Journal of Medical Ethics 21 (5): 265-269

Kohl M 1974 The morality of killing. Owen, London
Kohl M (ed) 1975 Beneficent euthanasia. Prometheus Books, New York
Kohner N, Henley A 2001 When a baby dies. Routledge, London
Kuhse H 1987 The sanctity of life doctrine in medicine. Oxford University Press, New York
Kuhse H, Singer P 1985 Should the baby live? Oxford University Press, Oxford
Kuhse H, Singer P (eds) 1999 Bioethics: an anthology. Blackwell, Oxford
Lamb D 1988 Down the slippery slope. In: Braine D, Lesser H Ethics, technology and medicine. Avebury Press, Aldershot
Landman W A, Henley L D 1998 Tensions in setting health care priorities for South Africa's children. Journal of Medical Ethics 24 (4): 268-273
Lee R, Morgan D (eds) 1989 Birthrights: law and ethics at the beginnings of life. Routledge, London
MacLachlan M, Dennis P, Lang H et al 1989 Do the professionals understand? In Brechin A, Walmsley J (eds) Making connections. Hodder and Stoughton, London
Martin A 2001 Scars of the NICU http://wwwcomeunity.com
Mason J K, McCall Smith R A 1999 Law and medical ethics. Butterworth, London
Mattison D 2001 Preventing prematurity. March of Dimes http://www.marchofdimes.com accessed 27.3.02
McCarthy C 2002 Fight for life. The Guardian [letters] 24 Apr: 9
McHaffie H E, Fowlie P W 1996 Life and death decisions. Hochland and Hochland Ltd, Hale
McMillan R C (ed) 1987 Euthanasia and the newborn. Kluwer, Dordrecht
McNaughton D 1989 Killing and letting die. In: De Cruz P, McNaughton D By what right? Studies in medicine, ethics and the law. Penrhos, Newcastle
MENCAP 2002 A life in the day www.mencap.org.uk
Mifflin P Challinor 2001 Jodie and Mary: Ethical and legal implications of separating conjoined twins. The Practising Midwife 4 (7): 48-49
Miller P 1996 Ethical issues in neonatal intensive care. In: Frith L (ed) Ethics and midwifery. Butterworth-Heinemann, Oxford
Mitchell R 1986 Ethical issues in neonatal nursing. In: Angelini D J, Knapp C N F, Hankins LC et al (eds) Obstetrics. Prentice Hall, Pearson Education, Harlow
Mittler P 1988 Quality of life for people with disabilities. In: Fairburn G, Fairburn S Ethical issues in caring. Avebury Press, Aldershot
Mittler P, Mittler H (eds) 1994 Innovation in family support for people with learning disabilities. Lisieux Hall, Chorley
Montgomery J 1997 Health care law. Oxford University Press, Oxford
Moorhead J 2002 An everyday tragedy. The Guardian 10th Jan: 14
Moreno J D 1999 Ethics consultation as moral engagement. In: Kuhse H, Singer P Bioethics: an anthology. Blackwell, Oxford
Morrison M F, Demichele M D 1997 How culture and religion affect attitudes towards medical futility. In: Zucker M B, Zucker H D (eds) Medical futility. Cambridge University Press, Cambridge
Mutch E 1997 Stress and parenting a disabled child. Social Work Monographs, Norwich
Newson E, Davis J 1994 Supporting the siblings of children with autism and related developmental disorders. In: Mittler P, Mittler H Innovation in family support for people with learning disabilities. Lisieux Hall, Chorley
Olshansky S 1962 Chronic sorrow: a response to having a mentally defective child. Social Casework 43: 190-193
Patterson F, Gordon W 1994 The case for the personhood of gorillas. In: Cavalieri P, Singer P (eds) The great ape project. St Martin's Press, New York
Pence G E (ed) 1995 Classic cases in medical ethics. McGraw Hill, New York

Pritchard J 1996 Ethical decision making and the positive use of codes. In: Frith L (ed) Ethics and midwifery. Butterworth-Heinemann, Oxford
Purcell C 1997 Withdrawing treatment from a critically ill child. Intensive and Critical Care Nursing 13 (2): 103-107
Quine L, Pahl J 1985 Examining the causes of stress in families with severely mentally handicapped children. British Journal of Social Work 15 (5): 501-517
Rachels J 1986 The end of life. Oxford University Press, Oxford
Rawls J 1973 A theory of justice. Oxford University Press, Oxford
Redshaw M 2002 A new kind of nurse. information@bliss.org.uk
Richardson A 1989 If you love him, let him go. In: Brechin A, Walmsley J Making connections. Hodder and Stoughton, London
Risdon R 2002. In: Heathcote E Mothers who kill. Independent on Sunday 21 Apr: 19
Robertson J 1998 Involuntary euthanasia of defective newborns. In: Pence G E (ed) Classic works in medical ethics. McGraw Hill, Boston MA
Robinson C, Stalker K 1993 Patterns of provision of respite care and the Children Act. British Journal of Social Work 23: 45-63
Sabbeth, Leventhal 1984 Marital adjustments to chronic childhood illness. Paediatrics 73: 927
Sainsbury K 1998 Whose life is it? The Guardian 15th Jul: 6
Seedhouse D 1995 Why bioethicists have nothing useful to say about health care rationing. Journal of Medical Ethics 21 (5): 288-291
Shaw A B 1999 In defence of ageism. In: Kuhse H, Singer P (eds) Bioethics: an anthology. Blackwell, Oxford
Shinwell E S 2000 Early postnatal dexamethasone treatment and incidence of cerebral palsy. Archives of Diseases in Childhood (Fetal and Neonatal Edition) 83: F177-F181
Sim J 1997 Ethical decision making in therapy practice. Butterworth-Heinemann, Oxford
Simeonsson R J, Bailey D B 1986 Siblings of handicapped children. In: Gallagher J J, Vietze P M (eds) Families of handicapped persons. Brookes, Baltimore
Simons J 2002. In: Smith D Despair that marks the death of a child. Daily Express 8th Jan: 3
Singer P (ed) 1993 A companion to ethics. Blackwell, Oxford
Singer P 1996 Rethinking life and death. St Martin's Griffin, New York
Singleton J, McLaren S 1995 Ethical foundations of healthcare. Mosby: London
Sloper P A, Turner S 1993 Risk and resistance factors in the adaptation of parents of children with severe physical disabilities. Journal of Child Psychology and Psychiatry 34:167-188
Sommerfield J 2001 Born too soon: prematurity rising. http://www.msnbc.com/new
Sone K 1995 Kith and kids. Community Care 1065: 16-17
Stinson R, Stinson P 1981 On the death of a baby. Journal of Medical Ethics 9 (1): 18
Summers S 2002 Special deliveries. The Observer (Magazine supplement) 17th Mar: 35-41
Sweet B R 1984 Sweet and Cape's obstetric care. Wiley and Son, Chichester
Sykes M Pro Choice Views. http://www.prochoice.about.com/newsissues
Thomasina D C, Kushner T 1996 Birth to death: science and bioethics. Cambridge University Press, Cambridge
Tooley M 1986 Abortion and infanticide. In: Singer P (ed) Applied ethics. Oxford University Press, Oxford
Tritt S, Esses L 1998 Psychological adaptation of siblings of children with chronic medical illness. American Journal of Orthopsychiatry 158: 211-220
Tyson J 1995 Evidence-based ethics and the care of premature infants. The Future of Children 5 (1): 1-14

Versluys Z, De Leeuw R 1995 A Dutch report on the ethics of neonatal care. Journal of Medical Ethics 21 (1): 14-16
Walters J W 1988 Approaches to ethical decision making in the neonatal intensive care unit. American Journal of the Disabled Child 142: 825-830
Watkins A 2002 Mr Brown's budget speech was an insult. The Independent on Sunday 21st Apr: 23
Wells C 1989 Marginal children. In: Lee R, Morgan D Birthrights: law and ethics at the beginnings of life. Routledge, London
Woodrum D E 2000 Neonatal ICU issues: ethical topics in medicine. University of Washington School of Medicine, Washington DC http://eduserv.hscer.washington.edu/bioethics/topics/nicu.html
Wyatt J, Spencer A 1992 Survival of the weakest. Christian Medical Fellowship, London
Zucker M B, Zucker H D (eds) 1997 Medical futility. Cambridge University Press, Cambridge

FURTHER READING

Adams J A 1996 The critically ill neonate. In: Thomasina D C, Kushner T Birth to death: science and bioethics. Cambridge University Press, Cambridge
Culyer A J 1998 Need: is a consensus possible? Journal of Medical Ethics 24 (2): 77-80
Cunningham F G, MacDonald P C, Norman F G et al (eds) 1997 Perinatal and neonatal nursing. Blackwell Scientific Publications, Oxford
De Cruz P, McNaughton D 1989 By what right? Studies in medicine, ethics and law. Penrhos, Newcastle
Goldworth A 1996 Medical technology and the child. In: Thomasina D C, Kushner T Birth to death: science and bioethics. Cambridge University Press, Cambridge
Grobstein C 1981 From chance to purpose. Addison Wesley, Reading MA
Hoare P, Harris M, Jackson P et al 1998 A community survey of children with severe intellectual disability and their families: psychological adjustment, carer distress and the effect of respite care. Journal of Intellectual Disability Research 42 (3): 218-227
Jenkins R 1995 The law and the midwife. Blackwell, Oxford
McMahan J 1996 Cognitive disability, misfortune and justice. Philosophy and Public Affairs 25 (7): 3-34
Sklansky M 2001 Neonatal euthanasia: moral considerations and criminal liability. Journal of Medical Ethics 27 (1): 5-11
Solomon S D 1995 Suffer the little children. Technology Review 98 10 Apr: 42
Steele A, Hawkey M 1994 Moral dimensions. Nursing Times 90 (37): 58
Telfer F 1994 A matter of ethics. Nursing Times 90 (28): 58

Index

A

B

C

D

T

V

W